T0251422

Vitamin Intake and Health

Vitamin Intake and Health

A Scientific Review

Suzanne K. Gaby
Adrianne Bendich
Vishwa N. Singh
Lawrence J. Machlin

Department of Clinical Nutrition
Hoffmann-La Roche, Inc.
Nutley, New Jersey

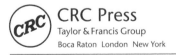

CRC Press
Taylor & Francis Group
Boca Raton London New York

CRC Press is an imprint of the
Taylor & Francis Group, an **informa** business

Foreword

Vitamin Intake and Health deals with one of the most fundamental, controversial, and potentially most important current issues in human nutrition. It concerns the question of suboptimal nutrient intake in apparently healthy individuals and the possible beneficial effects of optimal intake on overall health and longevity. It is indeed a scientific treatise with a wealth of analytical detail describing biochemical function and physiological effects of the clinically important vitamins, as well as survey data about relationships of disease to nutritional status. Replete with figures, summary tables, and references, the book provides a valuable source of concise information. One of the recurring themes is the problem of assessing nutritional status in individuals. Because of uncertainties in defining normal nutritional status, much of the currently available information is based on epidemiological methods involving rather large populations and crude estimates of food and nutrient intake. Investigators are often obliged to content themselves with making observations as to what people are and what they actually do under natural conditions rather than what might be best. In many situations, an assumption is made regarding health without establishing the absence of disease. There has been a tendency to confuse "normal" as in a normal, bell-shaped curve, with the word meaning normal health.

One must assume, however sadly, that fully satisfactory nutrition information will not be available until standardized assessment methods are developed and applied longitudinally in humans, as in the Framingham study of dietary lipids and heart disease. It would obviously be a task of monumental dimensions to evaluate the long-term health effects of all known essential nutrients, although this would clearly be a desirable goal. Meanwhile, for many years to come, it will probably be necessary to rely on reference standards such as the Recommended Dietary Allowances (RDA) to estimate the adequacy of dietary intake of populations in epidemiological studies. In spite of criticisms of the RDAs, it must be noted that they serve a very worthwhile purpose and will undoubtedly continue to serve as a valuable point of reference in the foreseeable future. This book should help bring into sharper focus an aspect of decision-making that may help establish clearer guidelines for nutrient intake, namely, optimal long-term health and longevity. Thus, it raises serious questions, perhaps indirectly, about the basic concept, principles, and use of the RDA.

It is widely acknowledged that RDAs were originally designed for use in national planning and for making estimates of average daily nutritional requirements of population groups made up of healthy individuals. However, it is becoming increasingly difficult to confine the use of the RDAs to their original purpose. As emphasized in the opening pages of this book, one can never be sure from survey data if individuals with the lowest nutrient intakes are indeed those with the lowest requirement. More importantly, one cannot be sure that they are indeed *healthy*. It is becoming more and more apparent that "healthy normal people" are an ideal concept rather than a practical reality. As a result, special attention must now be directed at subpopulations of millions of people who make up our complex society. In the aging population alone, approximately 80% suffer from at least one chronic disease. Examples of other factors that may impose deviations from "normal" requirements are heterozygous genetic disorders, the widespread use of prescription and nonprescription drugs, toxic environmental exposure, alcoholism, and other behavioral abnormalities. One may well ask, "Who is healthy; what is the definition of health?" It is probably no longer justifiable to single out for special consideration only such time-honored groups as pregnant women and growing children. Nor is it unreasonable to ask if diet modification or vitamin supplementation in apparently healthy individuals might prolong symptom-free intervals in chronic disease states, or prevent the onset of cancer, atherosclerosis, and certain other major illnesses.

For the first time in the history of the RDA, the most recent recommendations acknowledge that people who smoke have a higher requirement for vitamin C than nonsmokers. It is therefore implicit in this recommendation that recognition is now being given to long-term effects of nutrient intake, as opposed to classical concepts of acute deficiency disorders and minimum requirements. This recommendation, furthermore, gives tacit approval for the use of an entirely different set of end points to determine an optimal state of nutrition. Thus, in the case of smokers and vitamin C, an important factor in future considerations of nutrient requirements will be the amount necessary to minimize the risk of cancer and heart disease in a population at risk; a new dimension has been added to the assessment variables. In the case of vitamin A and carotenoids it may be necessary to consider the prevention of various forms of cancer as well as immunological compromise. In the case of folic acid it may be necessary to allow an amount sufficient to prevent the occurrence and/or recurrence of neural tube defects. The latter example seems particularly relevant, and indeed poignant, since it reflects a state of health that is adequate for conception to occur, yet inadequate for fetal requirements at a crucial stage of development. Evidence is cited that simply ingesting an inexpensive multiple-vitamin supplement during the period just before and just after conception dramatically and significantly reduces the incidence of neural tube defects at the time of parturition.

This is just one example of this book's orientation toward optimal nutrient intakes. The basic message is twofold and of the utmost significance: first, there are subpopulations with needs that may differ from those of the general population, and second, long-range benefits may be derived from special diets and/or supplements in individuals who might not otherwise exhibit the conventionally recognizable clinical manifestations of deficiency. Furthermore, the second part of the message implies clearly that there may be benefits of vitamin supplementation that are quite different from the purposes for which the vitamin was originally recognized. This book, with its wide-ranging scholarly analyses and exhaustive literature review, should provide food for thought to nutrition scientists for many years to come.

C. E. Butterworth, Jr., M.D.
General Foods Professor of Nutrition Sciences
Associate Dean for Research
Department of Nutrition Sciences
The University of Alabama at Birmingham
Birmingham, Alabama

Preface

The traditional concern of nutritionists and dietitians has been to ensure the consumption of vitamins in quantities sufficient to prevent deficiency diseases. A growing body of evidence suggests, however, that intakes of certain vitamins above usually recommended levels may help protect against the development of a number of chronic diseases. This book critically evaluates research in this area. The analysis focuses primarily on human studies, covering both studies of supplementation and epidemiological studies associating dietary intake of vitamins with health status. The benefits of vitamin supplementation in the treatment of frank deficiency diseases, malabsorption syndromes, and certain inborn errors of metabolism are well recognized, and are not covered in detail.

The introduction discusses nutrient intake and status in the United States and general mechanisms of vitamin function. Chapters 2 through 10 review the health implications of the status and/or the intake of individual vitamins, while Chapter 11 reviews studies using multivitamin supplements. Each chapter has an extensive list of references, and summary tables appear throughout the text.

Suzanne K. Gaby
Adrianne Bendich
Vishwa N. Singh
Lawrence J. Machlin

Contents

Vitamin Intake and Health

1

General Introduction

I. VITAMIN REQUIREMENTS

Vitamins are essential organic micronutrients which cause deficiency disorders when intake is inadequate (Table 1). In the past, dietary vitamin levels that can prevent deficiency symptoms and maintain a reserve body pool have generally been considered adequate. However, current research suggests that recommended levels of intake based on these criteria may not provide for optimal health benefits under all circumstances. The Recommended Daily Dietary Allowances are based on the estimated needs of "most healthy people" without a precise definition of whom this population includes.

Many individuals may have health problems, habits, or living situations in which chronic or periodic intake of vitamins should exceed the ordinary requirement. Examples of those who may have increased vitamin requirements include: cigarette smokers, oral contraceptive users, laxative abusers, alcohol abusers, habitual users of analgesics for chronic disease, and individuals with specific disorders of the gastrointestinal tract.

A. Marginal Deficiencies

A marginal, or subclinical, vitamin deficiency describes a condition in which vitamin status is poor (depleted reserves or localized deficiencies)

1

Table 1.   Some Vitamin Deficiency Diseases and Symptoms

Vitamin	Deficiency disease/major symptoms
A (retinol)	Xerophthalmia, night blindness, blindness
Thiamin (B_1)	Beriberi,numbness, muscle weakness, cardiac disturbance; Wernicke's encephalopathy, polyneuropathy
Riboflavin (B_2)	Glossitis, dermatitis, cheilosis
Niacin	Pellagra, dermatitis, diarrhea, mental disturbance
B_6 (pyridoxine)	Macrocytic anemia, dermatitis, depression, convulsions
B_{12} (cobalamin)	Macrocytic anemia, peripheral neuritis, spinal cord degeneration
Biotin	Dermatitis, anorexia, muscular pain, burning/tingling sensations
Pantothenic acid	Nervous and intestinal disorders
C (ascorbic acid)	Scurvy, sore gums, capillary bleeding
D (cholecalciferol)	Rickets, bone deformities, tetany
E (tocopherol)	Neuromuscular dysfunction, hemolytic anemia
Folic acid (folate, folacin)	Anemia, macrocytic anemia
K (phylloquinone)	Decreased clotting, bleeding

but no overt symptoms of a deficiency are present.   While the absence of obvious malnutrition was previously considered to represent good nutrition, the importance of preventing functional metabolic disturbances that can evolve into overt clinical symptoms has been recognized (Pietrzik, 1985). In a U.S. study, subclinical vitamin deficiencies were reported in groups of schoolchildren, elderly people, neonates, and mothers at time of delivery (Baker and Frank, 1985). It has been theorized that chronic marginal vitamin deficiencies may reduce resistance to environmental toxins and carcinogens. It has also been suggested that chronic marginal micronutrient status deleteriously affects physical performance (Powers et al., 1985, Vanderbeek et al., 1985), immune function, and mental behavior (Buzina, 1981).

The problem of recognizing subclinical vitamin deficiencies is confounded in the case of vitamin A, where severely depressed liver stores of the vitamin may be associated with normal plasma retinol, retinol binding protein (RBP), and RBP saturation indices (Amedee–Manesme et al., 1984). A test aimed specifically at revealing inadequate vitamin A status (relative dose response) confirmed that serum level analyses of the vitamin were not sufficient to recognize the inadequate vitamin A status of some

Brazilian children (Flores et al., 1984). A study examining French children with liver disease showed that, in spite of apparently normal eyes, conjunctival cells indicated a preclinical vitamin A deficiency (Amedee–Manesme et al., 1988). The significance of unrecognized subclinical vitamin A status is highlighted by the finding that vitamin A supplementation of a marginally deficient population resulted in significant vision improvement (Wilson et al., 1985). These are some examples of the need to identify and correct subclinical nutrient deficiencies.

II. U.S. RECOMMENDED DAILY ALLOWANCES AND TYPICAL NUTRIENT INTAKES

The Recommended Dietary Allowances (RDA) of the National Academy of Sciences are intended as guidelines for preventing deficiencies and maintaining reasonable reserves among most healthy people. For most nutrients, data on the intake necessary to prevent signs of a deficiency disease in young, healthy adults is extrapolated to the general population. To establish an RDA, a large margin of safety is added to the estimate, with more or less precision. The RDAs are also intended to be related to the nutrient status of population groups, not individuals, who may differ greatly (even when healthy) in their nutrient needs. The U.S. RDA is a simplified reference for labeling purposes, and is designed for individuals over 4 years of age (excluding pregnant and lactating women, who are considered separately). The U.S. RDA is based on the 1968 RDA and designed to include the highest RDA in any of the age/sex subgroups. Some of the U.S. RDAs are shown in Table 2.

Survey data indicate that substantial proportions of population subgroups are not meeting RDA levels of nutrient intake. Because the RDAs address the adequacy of intake in populations, this does not mean that individuals are necessarily at risk for deficiencies. By the same token, survey data do not determine whether or not those individuals with the lowest intakes are indeed those with the lowest requirements. It is a common misuse of the RDAs to try to evaluate the adequacy of individuals' diets by comparison with these population guidelines. Nevertheless, short of biochemical analyses and medical examination, an evaluation of nutritional status is difficult to make without resorting to the RDA reference points.

Although nutrient intakes lower than RDA levels are, by definition sufficient to prevent deficiency in some segments of the U.S. population, "the risk of having an inadequate intake increases to the extent that intake is less than the level recommended as safe" (Committee on Dietary Allowances, 1980).

Table 2. United States Recommended Daily Allowances of Vitamins

Vitamin	Children under 4 yrs	Adults and children 4 or more yrs	Pregnant or lactating women
Vitamin A	2500 IU	5000 IU	8000 IU
Vitamin D	400 IU	400 IU	400 IU
Vitamin E	10 IU	30 IU	30 IU
Vitamin C	40 mg	60 mg	60 mg
Folic acid	200 μg	400 μg	800 μg
Thiamin	0.7 mg	1.5 mg	1.7 mg
Riboflavin	0.8 mg	1.7 mg	2.0 mg
Niacin	9 mg	20 mg	20 mg
Vitamin B_6	0.7 mg	2.0 mg	2.5 mg
Vitamin B_{12}	3 μg	6 μg	8 μg
Biotin	0.15 mg	0.3 mg	0.3 mg
Pantothenic acid	5 mg	10 mg	10 mg

Source: Food and Drug Administration, 1973.

Many Americans do, in fact, have poor intakes of some nutrients. In the 1985 Nationwide Food Consumption Survey, for instance, the mean intake of folacin was less than half of the RDA for women (aged 19–50 years) in all income categories (U.S. Department of Agriculture, 1985). Low intakes of vitamin B_6 were also reported. Whereas *average* values of nutrient consumption suggest that vitamin intake is adequate for an entire population, individual intakes may be at unacceptable levels. Forty–one percent of the women surveyed were consuming less than 70% of the RDA for vitamin E; only 2% were consuming at least the RDA for folacin, and only 6% the RDA for vitamin B_6 (Table 3). It remains to be seen whether the RDA level has been arbitrarily set too high, or if dietary intakes of these nutrients should be increased. Table 4 shows the proportion of individuals representative of the general population with intakes of some vitamins below 70 and 100% of the RDA.

Poor nutrient status in significant numbers of people is not surprising given that the American diet tends to be high in fat and low in fiber (i.e., foods high in calories and comparatively low in essential nutrients). The Second National Health and Nutrition Examination Survey (NHANES II) found that only 21% of respondents (blacks and whites of both sexes) ate any fruit or vegetable high in vitamin A within a 24–hour period, and only 28% consumed a high–vitamin C fruit or vegetable (Patterson and Block,

Table 3. Percentage of Women Aged 19–50 Years with Selected Levels of Nutrient Intake: 1985

Vitamin	Percent of RDA[a]	
	Less than 100%	Less than 70%
Vitamin A	54	37
Thiamin	53	21
Riboflavin	50	22
Niacin	33	11
Vitamin B6	94	73
Vitamin B12	40	19
Folic acid	98	87
Ascorbic acid	47	28
Vitamin E	70	41

[a]Numbers are rounded to the nearest percentage point. Based on 4 nonconsecutive days.
Source: USDA (1985), Nationwide Food Consumption Survey, Continuing Survey of Food Intakes by Individuals.

Table 4. Percentage of Individuals with Selected Levels of Nutrient Intake

Vitamin	Percent of RDA[a]	
	Less than 100%	Less than 70%
Vitamin A	50	31
Thiamine	45	17
Riboflavin	34	12
Niacin	33	9
Vitamin B6	80	51
Vitamin B12	34	15
Ascorbic acid	41	26

[a]Numbers are rounded to the nearest percentage point.
Source: Pao and Mickle (1981), from the USDA Nationwide Food Consumption Survey.

1988). On the day reported, only 59% ate any fruit of any kind (Patterson and Block, 1988).

In addition to the potential for population groups to fail to meet the RDA levels of nutrient intakes, a number of population subgroups are at risk of poor nutrient status due to increased requirements (Table 5). Table 5 is not intended to imply that 100% of the U.S. population is at risk of inadequate vitamin status. Clearly, many individuals would fall into more than one subgroup, e.g., adolescents who drink and smoke. Nevertheless, there are substantial numbers of people who would be considered at risk.

III. GROUPS AT RISK OF POOR VITAMIN STATUS

A. Smokers

Approximately one–third of American adults smoke cigarettes. Smoking is associated with an increased risk of cancer, cardiovascular disease, and chronic lung disease. Smokers have also been found to have a poorer status of a number of micronutrients than nonsmokers. Smokers tend to have lower blood levels of β–carotene (Witter et al., 1982; Chow et al., 1986; Aoki et al., 1987; Gerster, 1987) and pyridoxal–5'–phosphate (the active form of vitamin B6) (Serfontein et al., 1986). People who smoke also appear to have an increased requirement for vitamin C (Pelletier, 1970; Hornig and Glatthaar, 1985) and were found to have significantly lower levels of vitamin E in lung alveolar fluid (Pacht et al., 1986) in comparison with nonsmokers. These reduced nutrient levels may contribute to the health risks associated with smoking.

B. Dieters

Eating behavior, particularly diets that omit or severely restrict whole categories of foods, can have serious negative impact on micronutrient status. Diets that eliminate all animal foods provide almost no vitamin B12, and have also been associated with cases of rickets (vitamin D deficiency) (Dwyer et al., 1979) and other vitamin deficiencies (Zmora et al., 1979) in children. Skipping meals and dieting to lose weight frequently compromise micronutrient intake. In general it is extremely difficult to meet all of the requirements for micronutrients at intakes of less than 1200 calories per day. An analysis of 11 published reducing diets showed that none provided 100% of the U.S. RDA for representative vitamins (Fisher and Lachance, 1985).

C. Oral Contraceptive Users and Users of Other Medications

The use of oral contraceptive agents (OCA) is associated with decreased plasma levels of some vitamins. Although OCA users and nonusers were

Table 5.   Selected Groups at Risk of Poor Vitamin Status in the U.S. Population

Group	Estimated number as % of population	Nutrients[a]
Adolescents (10–19 years)	14.6[b]	Folate, vitamin A
Alcohol users—3 or more drinks/week	22*[b]	Thiamin, vitamins A, B6, and D, folate, β–carotene
Cigarette smokers	28.6**[b]	Vitamins B6, E, & C, β–carotene, folate
Diabetics	4.6[c]	Vitamins B6, C and D
Dieters	20[d]	Potentially any or all
Elderly (≥65 yrs)	12.1[e]	Vitamins C and D, folate
Oral contraceptive users	10.4***[c]	Vitamin B6, folate, β–carotene
Pregnant women[f]	3.9***[b]	All, especially folate
Strict vegetarians[g]	>0.9	Vitamins B12 and D

*Percentage of population ≥ 18 years.

**Percentage of population ≥ 20 years.

***Percentage of women ≥ 16 years.

[a]References are cited in the text.

[b]U.S. Bureau of the Census (1987).

[c]The Surgeon General's Report on Nutrition and Health (1988); based on an estimated 11 million diabetic individuals in a total population of 240 million, and 10 million women taking oral contraceptives in a female population (over the age of 15) of 96 million.

[d]Fisher and Lachance (1985)

[e]Projected for 1990, *Current Population Reports*, Series P–25, no. 704, "Projections of the Population of the United States: 1977–2050."

[f]Estimate based on the number of live births. The U.S. RDA is the same for pregnant and lactating women; in 1980–1981, 32.6% of infants were breast–fed 3 or more months (U.S. Bureau of the Census, 1987).

[g]Estimate for 1980, from Smith (1988).

found to have comparable nutrient intake, OCA users had lower plasma carotene and pyridoxal phosphate levels and lower red blood cell folate than nonusers (Prasad et al., 1975). OCA use is associated with an apparent increased requirement for vitamin B6 (Driskell et al., 1976). OCA users also have lower vitamin C levels (Rivers and Devine, 1972).

Many commonly used medications, including antibotics and antacids, are known to interfere with the absorption and/or metabolism of nutrients (Brin, 1978; Roe, 1985). For example, both aspirin and anticonvulsants can inhibit absorption of folate (Roe, 1974). This represents a particular problem because some medications (like antacids, aspirin and anticonvulsants) are taken chronically.

D. Alcohol Users

The regular use of alcohol can alter the metabolism of vitamin D (Lieber et al., 1987) and is associated with low serum levels of folate, thiamin, and vitamin B6 (Halsted and Heise, 1987). Low serum β–carotene concentrations were found in regular alcohol drinkers, with still lower levels seen in drinkers who smoke (Aoki et al., 1987). Alcoholics often have extremely low liver stores of vitamin A, even when blood levels of retinol are normal (Lieber et al., 1987). Ingestion of ethanol has been shown to interfere with intestinal absorption of vitamin C (Fazio et al., 1981). Impaired micronutrient metabolism has also been associated with other drugs of abuse (Lieber et al., 1987).

E. Adolescents

During periods of rapid growth, particularly during adolescence, high nutrient demands may not be met by a typical diet. Red blood cell folate was at a deficient level in 47.6% of a group of apparently healthy teenage girls in Alabama (Clark et al., 1987). In spite of normal blood measurements of vitamin A status, mean dietary vitamin A intake of black teenage males in Kentucky was only 36% of the U.S. RDA, and white teenage females consumed about 51% of the U.S. RDA of that nutrient (Lee, 1978). All groups of teens studied in Kentucky also had a high incidence of unacceptably low hemoglobin levels (Lee, 1978). Twelve percent of a group of adolescent girls in North Carolina consumed less than two–thirds of the RDA of vitamin A, but 20% had marginal serum vitamin A levels (Sumner et al., 1987). While nutrient demands are particularly high during puberty, eating habits may be particularly poor. This may be due in part to reducing diets.

F. Pregnant and Lactating Women

Increased nutritional requirements during pregnancy and lactation are universally acknowledged. Nonetheless, pregnant women may not be meeting these requirements and may be sacrificing their own nutritional status in maintaining the conceptus. Nutrient adequacy is critical during the first trimester of pregnancy. In 1981, however, only 79% of white mothers and 62% of black mothers received prenatal care during the first trimester of pregnancy (U.S. Dept. of Health and Human Services, 1984). Even with normal, healthy pregnancies, nearly one–fourth of women tested in one study were deficient in at least one essential nutrient at the time of delivery (Vobecky and Vobecky, 1988).

G. Elderly

Advanced age has been associated with marginal vitamin deficiencies in numerous studies (Kirsch and Bidlack, 1987). Many elderly people may not be adequately nourished owing to poor diet, dental problems, lack of mobility, reduced caloric needs (reducing micronutrient intake), drug/nutrient interactions, chronic illness, and economic restraints. Older individuals also may have difficulty digesting and/or absorbing nutrients; for example, one study reported that elderly subjects had a reduced ability (relative to younger subjects) to obtain folate from foods (Baker et al., 1978).

Since nutrient requirements for older people are primarily extrapolated from young subjects, it is unclear whether and to what extent nutrient needs increase with age. Alterations in metabolism may explain declines in nutrient status in aging well–nourished individuals. For example, platelet tocopherol (vitamin E) concentrations have been found to decrease significantly with age, although plasma levels remain unchanged (Vatassery et al., 1983).

Thus, for numerous reasons the elderly represent a large (and expanding) segment of the population that is at risk for nutritional problems. It has been suggested that unrecognized scurvy may even be common among the elderly (Connelly et al., 1982). A comparison of mean plasma vitamin C levels in young adults and elderly subjects showed that the older group had less than half the blood concentration of ascorbic acid found in the younger group (Schorah, 1978). A very high incidence of vitamin B_6 deficiency was noted among institutionalized elderly subjects in France (Guilland et al., 1984). Otherwise adequately nourished older people in New Mexico were found to have a poor vitamin D intake (Garry et al., 1982).

H. Premature Infants

Low-birth-weight (LBW) infants (less than 5 1/2 lb or 2500g) are at risk for serious health problems and increased mortality. In 1985 there were 6.8 LBW infants per 100 births in the United States (5.6% among whites, 12.4% among blacks) (Centers for Disease Control, 1988). Premature infants have been found to have low plasma vitamin C levels (Heinonen et al., 1986), low vitamin A status (Shenai et al., 1981), and a proneness to vitamin E deficiency (*Nutrition Reviews,* 1986). Because small infants can ingest only limited amounts of milk, and because their nutrient reserves are minimal at best, vitamin supplementation is necessary for this population. The nutrients of particular concern are the fat-soluble vitamins, folic acid, vitamin C (Heird and Cooper, 1988) and vitamin B_6 (Orzalesi, 1982).

I. Diabetics

About 11 million Americans have diabetes (Surgeon General's Report, 1988). Diabetic individuals may be at risk of marginal thiamin deficiency (Saito et al., 1987) and low status of other B vitamins, ascorbic acid, and vitamin D (Mooradian and Morley, 1987). It has been theorized that micronutrient supplementation may improve glucose tolerance and other abnormalities of metabolism in diabetes (McCarty and Rubin, 1984).

IV. MECHANISMS OF VITAMIN ACTION

A. The Coenzyme Function of Vitamins

Enzymes catalyze most of the metabolic processes in the body. The major portion of an enzyme, the apoenzyme, is mainly composed of protein and is synthesized de novo. In order for most enzymes to function they require coenzymes, such as the water-soluble vitamins and vitamin K, and/or cofactors, which are either vitamins or minerals.

Because the body can synthesize apoenzymes, the limiting factor affecting enzyme activity is the availability of coenzymes and cofactors which must be consumed in the diet. The role of certain vitamins as coenzymes has traditionally been the focus of vitamin research. The coenzyme and cofactor roles for the water-soluble vitamins are certainly of critical importance. For instance, vitamin B_6 is required in over half of the body's enzyme reactions, including most reactions involving amino acids. Folic acid is necessary for the activity of enzymes involved in DNA synthesis. Some of the classical vitamin deficiency disease symptoms are the result of inadequate coenzyme levels. Once the apoenzyme is associated with its coenzyme, further increases in the coenzyme concentration do not increase enzyme activity. Thus one can saturate the system, and this has led to the perception that higher intakes of vitamins with coenzyme function serve no useful purpose. However, as more is learned about the noncoenzyme functions of the vitamins that serve as coenzymes, this hypothesis has been revised. In addition, a number of vitamins have functions that are not linked to enzymatic activities. Vitamins A and E and the prohormone vitamin D do not function as cofactors or coenzymes.

The recognition of other functions of vitamins, such as antioxidant activity, has expanded our views of vitamin function.

B. Antioxidant Function

1. Oxidation and Free Radical Damage

Although oxygen is absolutely essential to metabolism, it can play a role in damaging cells. Most of the damaging effects of oxygen result from oxygen–containing free radicals. Free radicals contain atoms with one or more unpaired electrons. A free radical is unstable and tends toward stabilization by pairing the electron; this can destabilize a neighboring molecule through the removal of one of its electrons. This sets up a chain reaction as each succeeding molecule is made reactive and then seeks to stabilize itself. During these reactions, free radical oxidative damage can destroy cells. The basic process may be compared to the damage done to food as it becomes rancid.

2. Antioxidants

The destructive chain reaction started by free radicals can be broken by antioxidants, which are converted by the process into harmless derivatives. Antioxidants help to maintain a stable internal environment in plants and animals. The body has many natural protective mechanisms to contain oxidative damage: (a) antioxidant nutrients such as β-carotene, vitamins C and E; (b) other small molecules with antioxidant properties, for example, glutathione and uric acid; and (c) enzymes such as superoxide dismutase and glutathione peroxidase.

3. Antioxidants, Free Radicals and Cancer

If free radical damage occurs in the nucleus of the cell and damages DNA, it can cause mutations (Saul et al., 1987; Totter, 1980). If certain segments of the DNA are affected it may initiate malignant change, potentially leading to cancer. Since antioxidants can protect cells from free radical damage, it is possible that antioxidants may protect against carcinogenic agents (for reviews, see Draper and Bird, 1984; Halliwell and Gutteridge, 1985; Vuillaume, 1987), a possibility that is under investigation in a number of well-controlled human studies.

4. Free Radicals and Cardiovascular Disease

The development of atherosclerosis, which can lead to arteriosclerosis and hypertension, begins with damage to arterial walls. There is a large body of evidence that free radicals can directly and indirectly cause substantial damage to vascular endothelial cells (Rubanyi, 1988). Platelets tend to aggregate at the site of injury, leading to the deposition of fibrin and lipids, which ultimately form an atherosclerotic plaque (for a review, see Hennig and Chow, 1988). Antioxidants, therefore, may also have a role in the prevention of cardiovascular disease.

5. The Antioxidant Vitamins

The antioxidant functions of vitamins C and E and of β–carotene are being widely investigated because there may be a connection between the amounts of these micronutrients consumed and the amount of oxidative damage leading to cancers and degenerative diseases (Ames, 1983). For optimum antioxidant activity in the body, these vitamins may be required in higher amounts than those needed to prevent deficiency symptoms.

REFERENCES

Amedee-Manesme, O., Anderson, D., and Olson, J. A. (1984). Relation of the relative dose response to liver concentrations of vitamin A in generally well–nourished surgical patients. *Am. J. Clin. Nutr.* 39:898–902.

Amedee-Manesme, O., Luzeau, R., Wittepen, J. R., Hanck, A., and Sommer, A. (1988). Impression cytology detects subclinical vitamin A deficiency. *Am. J. Clin. Nutr.* 47:875–878.

Ames, B. N. (1983). Dietary carcinogens and anticarcinogens: oxygen radicals and degenerative diseases. *Science 221*:1256–1264.

Aoki, K., Ito, Y., Sasaki, R., Ohtani, M., Hamajima, N., and Asano, A. (1987). Smoking, alcohol drinking and serum carotenoids levels. *Jpn. J. Cancer Res. (Gann) 78*:1049–1056.

Baker, H. and Frank, O. (1985). Sub-clinical vitamin deficits in various age groups. *Int. J. Vit. Nutr. Res. Suppl. 27*:47–59.

Baker, H., Jaslow, S. P., and Frank, O. (1978). Severe impairment of dietary folate utilization in the elderly. *J. Am. Geriatr. Soc. 26*:218–221.

Brin, M. (1978). Drugs and environmental chemicals in relation to vitamin needs. In *Nutrition and Drug Interrelations*, J. N. Hathcock and J. Coon (Eds.), Academic Press, New York; pp. 131–150.

Buzina, R. (1981). Marginal malnutrition and its functional consequences in industrialized societies. *Prog. Clin. Biol. Res. 77*:285–303.

Centers for Disease Control (1988). Progress toward achieving the 1990 objectives for pregnancy and infant health. *Morbid. Mortal. Wkly. Rep. 37*:405–408, 413.

Chow, C. K., Thacker, R. R., Changchit, C., Bridges, R. B., Rehm, S. R., Humble, J., and Turbek, J. (1986). Lower levels of vitamin C and carotenes in plasma of cigarette smokers. *J. Am. Coll. Nutr. 5*:305–312.

Clark, A. J., Mossholder, S., and Gates, R. (1987). Folacin status in adolescent females. *Am. J. Clin. Nutr. 46*:302–306.

Committee on Dietary Allowances, Food and Nutrition Board (1980). Recommended Dietary Allowances, 9th rev. ed. National Academy of Sciences, Washington, DC.

Connelly, T. J., Becker, A., and McDonald, J. W. (1982). Bachelor scurvy. *Int. J. Dermatol. 21*:209–211.

Draper, H. H. and Bird, R. P. (1984). Antioxidants and cancer. *J. Agri. Food Chem. 32*:433–435.

Driskell, J. A., Geders, J. M., and Urban, M. C. (1976). Vitamin B6 status of young men, women, and women using oral contraceptives. *J. Lab. Clin. Med. 87*:813–821.

Dwyer, J. T., Dietz, W. H., Hass, G., and Suskind, R. (1979). Risk of nutritional rickets among vegetarian children. *Am. J. Dis. Child. 133*: 134–140.

Fazio, V., Flint, D. M., and Wahlqvist, M. L. (1981). Acute effects of alcohol on plasma ascorbic acid in healthy subjects. *Am. J. Clin. Nutr. 34*:2394–2396.

Fisher, M. C. and Lachance, P. A. (1985). Nutrition evaluation of published weight–reducing diets. *J. Am. Diet. Assoc. 85*:450–454.

Flores, H., Campos, F., Araujo, C. R. C., and Underwood, B. A. (1984). Assessment of marginal vitamin A deficiency in Brazilian children using the relative dose response procedure. *Am. J. Clin. Nutr. 40*:1281–1289.

Garry, P. J., Goodwin, J. S., Hunt, W. C., Hooper, E. M., and Leonard, A. G. (1982). Nutritional status in a healthy elderly population: dietary and supplemental intakes. *Am. J. Clin. Nutr. 36*:319–331.

Gerster, H. (1987). Beta–carotene and smoking. *J. Nutr. Growth Cancer 4*:45–49.

Guilland, J. C., Bereksi–Reguig, B., Lequeu, B., Moreau, D., and Klepping, J. (1984). Evaluation of pyridoxine intake and pyridoxine status among aged institutionalised people. *Int. J. Vit. Nutr. Res. 54*:185–193.

Halliwell, B. and Gutteridge, J. M. C. (1985). *Free Radicals in Biology and Medicine.* Clarendon Press, Oxford.

Halsted, C. H. and Heise, C. (1987). Ethanol and vitamin metabolism. *Pharmacol. Ther. 34*:453–464.

Heinonen, K., Mononen, I., Mononen, T., Parviainen, M., Penttila, I., and Launiala, K. (1986). Plasma vitamin C levels are low in premature infants fed human milk. *Am. J. Clin. Nutr. 43*:923–924.

Heird, W. C. and Cooper, A. (1988). Nutrition in infants and children. In *Modern Nutrition in Health and Disease*, 7th ed., M. E. Shils, and V. R.Young, Eds. Lea & Febiger, Philadelphia, pp. 944–968.

Hennig, B. and Chow, C. K. (1988). Lipid peroxidation and endothelial cell injury: implications in atherosclerosis. *Free Rad. Biol. Med. 4*:99–106.

Hornig, D. H. and Glatthaar, B. E. (1985). Vitamin C and smoking: increased requirement of smokers. *Int. J. Vit. Nutr. Res. Suppl. 27*:139–155.

Kirsch, A. and Bidlack, W. R. (1987). Nutrition and the elderly: vitamin status and efficacy of supplementation. *Nutrition 3*:305–314.

Lee, C. J. (1978). Nutritional status of selected teenagers in Kentucky. *Am. J. Clin. Nutr. 31*:1453–1464.

Lieber, C. S., Baraona, E., Leo, M. A., and Garro, A. (1987). Metabolism and metabolic effects of ethanol, including interaction with drugs, carcinogens and nutrition. *Mutat. Res. 186*:201–233.

McCarty, M. F. and Rubin, E. J. (1984). Rationales for micronutrient supplementation in diabetes. *Med. Hypotheses 13*:139–151.

Mooradian, A. D. and Morley, J. E. (1987). Micronutrient status in diabetes mellitus. *Am. J. Clin. Nutr. 45*:877–895.

Nutrition Reviews (1986). Vitamin E status of premature infants. *Nutr. Rev. 44*:166–167.

Orzalesi, M. (1982). Do breast and bottle fed babies require vitamin supplements? *Acta. Paediatr. Scand. Suppl. 299*:77–82.

Pacht, E. R., Kaseki, H., Mohammed, J. R., Cornwell, D. G., and Davis, W. B. (1986). Deficiency of vitamin E in the alveolar fluid of cigarette smokers: influence on alveolar macrophage cytotoxicity. *J. Clin. Invest. 77*:789–796.

Pao, E. M. and Mickle, S. J. (1981). Problem nutrients in the United States. *Food Technol. 35*:58–62, 64, 66–69, 79.

Patterson, B. H. and Block, G. (1988). Food choices and the cancer guidelines. *Am. J. Public Health 78*:282–286.

Pelletier, O. (1970). Vitamin C status of cigarette smokers and nonsmokers. *Am. J. Clin. Nutr. 23*:520–524.

Pietrzik, K. (1985). Concept of borderline vitamin deficiencies. *Int. J. Vit. Nutr. Res. Suppl. 27*:61–73

Powers, H. J., Bates, C. J., Lamb, W. H., Singh, J., Gelman, W., and Webb, E. (1985). Effects of a multivitamin and iron supplement on running performance in Gambian children. *Hum. Nutr. Clin. Nutr. 39*:427–437.

Prasad, A. S., Lei, K. Y., Oberleas, D., Moghissi, K. S., and Stryker, J. C. (1975). Effect of oral contraceptive agents on nutrients: II. Vitamins. *Am. J. Clin. Nutr. 28*:385–391.

Rivers, J. M. and Devine, M. M. (1972). Plasma ascorbic acid concentrations and oral contraceptives. *Am. J. Clin. Nutr. 25*:684–689.

Roe, D. (1974). Effects of drugs on nutrition. *Life Sci. 15*:1219–1234.

Roe, D. A. (1985). *Drug–Induced Nutritional Deficiencies*, 2nd ed. : AVI Publishing Co.,Westport, CT; pp. 1–87.

Rubanyi, G. M. (1988). Vascular effects of oxygen–derived free radicals. *Free Rad. Biol. Med. 4*:107–120.

Saito, N., Kimura, M., Kuchiba, A., and Itokawa, Y. (1987). Blood thiamine levels in outpatients with diabetes mellitus. *J. Nutr. Sci. Vitaminol. 33*:421–430.

Saul, R. L., Gee, P., and Ames, B. N. (1987). Free radicals, DNA damage, and aging. In *Modern Biological Theories of Aging*, H. R. Warner et al. Eds.. Raven Press, New York, pp. 113–129.

Serfontein, W. J., Ubbink, J. B., DeVilliers, L. S., and Becker, P. J. (1986). Depressed plasma pyridoxal–5'–phosphate levels in tobacco–smoking men. *Atherosclerosis 59*:341–346.

Schorah, C. J. (1978). Inappropriate vitamin C reserves: their frequency and significance in an urban population. In *The Importance of Vitamins to Health*, T. G. Taylor.(Ed.). MTP Press, Lancaster, England, pp. 61–72.

Shenai, J. P., Chytil, F., Jhaveri, A., and Stahlman, M. T. (1981). Plasma vitamin A and retinol–binding protein in premature and term neonates. *J. Pediatr. 99*:302–305.

Smith, M. V. (1988). Development of a quick reference guide to accommodate vegetarianism in diet therapy for multiple disease conditions. *Am. J. Clin. Nutr. 48*:906–909.

Sumner, S. K., Liebman, M., and Wakefield, L. M. (1987). Vitamin A status of adolescent girls. *Nutr. Rep. Int. 35*:423–431.

Surgeon General's Report (1988). *Surgeon General's Report on Nutrition and Health*. U. S. Dept. Health and Human Services, Washington, DC.

Thurnham, D. I. (1981). Red cell enzyme tests of vitamin status: do marginal deficiencies have any physiological significance? *Proc. Nutr. Soc. 40*:155–163.

Totter, J. R. (1980). Spontaneous cancer and its possible relationship to oxygen metabolism. *Proc. Natl. Acad. Sci. USA* 77:1763–1767.

U. S. Bureau of the Census (1987). *Statistical Abstract of the United States: 1988,* (108th ed.) Washington, DC.

U. S. Department of Agriculture, Human Nutrition Information Service (1985). Nationwide Food Consumption Survey, Continuing Survey of Food Intakes by Individuals. Women 19–50 Years and Their Children 1–5 Years, 4 Days. NFCS, CSFII Report No. 85–4.

U. S. Department of Health and Human Services (1984). *Health United States 1984.* Hyattsville, MD.

Vanderbeek, E. J., Vandokkum, W., Schrijver, J., and Hermus, R. J. J. (1985). Impact of marginal vitamin intake on physical performance in healthy young men. *Proc. Nutr. Soc. 44:*27A.

Vatassery, G. T., Johnson, G. J., and Krezowski, A. M. (1983). Changes in vitamin E concentrations in human plasma and platelets with age. *J. Am. Coll. Nutr. 4:*369–375.

Vobecky, J. S. and Vobecky, J. (1988). Vitamin status of women during pregnancy. In *Vitamins and Minerals in Pregnancy and Lactation,* H. Berger (Ed.) Nestle Nutrition Workshop Series, Vol. 16. Nestec Ltd., Vevey/Raven Press, New York, pp. 109–111.

Vuillaume, M. (1987). Reduced oxygen species, mutation, induction and cancer initiation. *Mutat. Res. 186:*43–72.

Wilson, D., Netto, O. B., Simao da Costa, A., Steiner, A., de Fatima Nunes Marucci, M., and Barbosa, M. C. (1985). Effect of vitamin A on visual accuracy. *Int. J. Vit. Nutr. Res. Suppl. 27:*117–120.

Witter, F. R., Blake, D. A., Baumgardner, R., Mellits, E. D., and Niebyl, J. R. (1982). Folate, carotene, and smoking. *Am. J. Obstet. Gynecol. 144:*857.

Zmora, E., Gorodischer, R., and Bar–Ziv, J. (1979). Multiple nutritional deficiencies in infants from a strict vegetarian community. *Am. J. Dis. Child. 133:*141–144.

2

Vitamin A

S. K. Gaby and A. Bendich

I. INTRODUCTION

Vitamin A (retinol) functions in reproduction, growth, the maintenance of skin and mucous membranes, and the visual process. Vitamin A is normally transported in the blood linked to a specific protein, retinol binding protein (RBP). Specific proteins on cell surfaces and within cells are also involved with intracellular transport of the vitamin.

Vitamin A is fat soluble and is primarily stored in the liver, where RBP is synthesized. In a well-nourished person, vitamin A stores are generally sufficient to last many months on a vitamin A-deficient diet before signs of deficiency appear. The initial symptoms of vitamin A deficiency are night blindness and keratinization of hair follicles. Continued deficiency leads to damage to eye tissue and irreversible blindness. The U.S. Recommended Daily Allowance (RDA) of vitamin A for adults is 5000 IU (1000 retinol equivalents). Rich dietary sources of retinol (preformed vitamin A) include dairy products, eggs, and organ meats. Some carotenoids (found in deep-yellow and dark-green vegetables) can be converted to vitamin A during digestion (see Chapter 3, "β-Carotene"). In the U.S. diet, approximately half of the vitamin A activity is derived from β-carotene and other carotenoids (Committee on Dietary Allowances, 1980).

II. HEALTH BENEFITS

A. Reduced Cancer Risk

1. Introduction

In epidemiological studies, a low intake of vitamin A has consistently been associated with increased risk of developing certain cancers (Kummet et al., 1983). However, the role of vitamin A in cancer etiology is confused by the failure, in many studies, to differentiate between preformed vitamin A (retinol) and carotenoids, which may have anticancer effects unrelated to their provitamin A function. Another difficulty in interpreting epidemiological data on vitamin A is that serum retinol and RBP do not necessarily reflect vitamin A status or intake. In addition, retinol status can be affected by protein malnutrition, liver disease, and infection.

There are several theorized mechanisms to explain cancer risk reduction by vitamin A. It is well established that vitamin A is required for the maintenance of epithelial tissues, where many cancers are seen. Vitamin A status must therefore be adequate to allow normal epithelial growth. Immune system function, including tumor surveillance, has also been shown in animal models to depend on sufficient levels of vitamin A (Moriguchi et al., 1985). In addition, vitamin A and retinoids (vitamin A derivatives) may directly influence gene expression (Sporn and Roberts, 1983).

2. Effect of Vitamin A on Cancer: Epidemiology

Even though there are problems in the relevance of these measurements, blood retinol and RBP levels are used as indices of vitamin A status in epidemiological studies. Low serum retinol has been reported in patients with both epithelial and nonepithelial tumors (Tyler et al., 1985). A prospective study suggests that blood retinol levels may decline as a result of progressing cancer (Wald et al., 1986). Low serum retinol levels have also been associated with an increased risk of subsequent cancer (Wald et al., 1980; Kark et al., 1981), though some reports have failed to confirm this (Peleg et al., 1984; Wald et al., 1986).

Patients who remained free of disease for 2 years after treatment for breast cancer had significantly higher RBP levels than those who suffered a reappearance of cancer (Mehta et al., 1987). A retrospective breast cancer case–control study evaluating food intake showed significantly less frequent vitamin A consumption in those who developed cancer (Katsouyanni et al., 1988). The association between intake and reduced risk was found for both retinol and β-carotene, although the separate associations were not as strong as for total vitamin A. In a similar study, however, no association was seen between dietary indices of β-carotene or retinol and cancer risk (Marubini et al., 1988).

Vitamin A intake does not appear to reduce the risk of bladder cancer (Tyler et al., 1986). In fact, high intake of the nutrient has been associated with increased bladder tumor recurrence (Michalek et al., 1987). In two studies, high intake of total vitamin A has been associated with an increased risk of prostate cancer (Heshmat et al., 1985; Kolonel et al., 1987). However, a high intake of high-fat animal foods, which have been associated with prostate cancer risk (Rotkin 1977) and which are rich sources of preformed vitamin A, may have resulted in a noncausal association in these studies (Mettlin et al., 1989). Additional studies have found no relationship between dietary retinol and prostrate cancer risk (Kaul et al., 1987), or reduced risk associated with high retinol intake (Ohno et al., 1988).

Although there is strong epidemiological evidence that β-carotene may reduce lung cancer risk, this association has not been clearly demonstrated for retinol intake (Ziegler et al., 1984; Samet et al., 1985; Bond et al., 1987; Humble et al., 1987). There was also no association seen between serum retinol or RBP and subsequent incidence of lung cancer (Friedman et al., 1986). In a number of studies, however, high intake of total vitamin A was associated with significantly lower risk of developing lung cancer (Humble et al., 1987). It may be (assuming a reasonable intake of β-carotene) that dietary retinol has a carotenoid–sparing effect that contributes to cancer risk reduction. However, the role of vitamin A in reducing lung cancer risk requires further examination. It was found, for example, that males from a group with lung cancer ate less liver, and fewer were found to have taken vitamin A supplements during the previous 20 years than matched controls without cancer (Gregor et al., 1980). A large, multicenter, National Cancer Institute–sponsored intervention trial is under way to explore the effects of both β-carotene and retinol on lung cancer incidence.

3.   Effect of Vitamin A on Precancerous Lesions:
     Intervention Trials

Oral leukoplakia is a lesion, occurring most commonly on the inside of the cheek (buccal mucosa), which can lead to oral cancer. People at risk of developing oral cancer also have localized genetic damage, indicated by the presence of micronucleated buccal mucosa cells. Serum levels of vitamin A were found to be lower in individuals with leukoplakias than in normals, and still lower in individuals with oral cancer (Wahi et al., 1962).

In a series of intervention trials with individuals at high risk for oral cancer due to betel nut and tobacco chewing, Stich et al. reported a decrease in micronucleated buccal cells after high-dose vitamin A supplementation (Stich et al., 1984a) and supplementation with vitamin A plus β-carotene (Stich et al., 1984b). In a similar group, supplementation with retinol prevented development of new oral leukoplakias and in some cases led to complete remission (Stich et al., 1988a). The beneficial effect appears to be strongest when retinol and β-carotene supplementation are combined (Stich et al., 1988b).

Among subjects from a group at high risk of developing esophageal cancer, and with a high incidence of precancerous esophageal lesions, raising blood retinol from low to high levels increased the likelihood of subjects having a histologically normal esophagus (Wahrendorf et al., 1988).

The influence of vitamin A intake and status on cancer etiology is a complicated area of investigation. Clinical intervention trials will be important in differentiating the effects of retinol from those of β-carotene.

B. Bronchopulmonary Dysplasia

Bronchopulmonary dysplasia (BPD) is a life-threatening condition seen in premature infants. BPD is thought to result from oxygen toxicity, artificial ventilation, and/or damage caused by other medical intervention such as endotracheal tubes (*Nutrition Reviews,* 1986). The respiratory tract changes present in BPD are similar to those seen in severe vitamin A deficiency (*Nutrition Reviews,* 1986). Premature infants commonly have low vitamin A stores, and a poor vitamin A status may interfere with the ability of lung tissue to repair the injury associated with BPD (Shenai et al., 1985).

Premature infants who develop BPD tend to have lower plasma retinol concentrations than those who do not. A significant proportion of these infants may have levels approaching the deficiency range (Hustead et al., 1984; Shenai et al., 1985).

High-dose supplementation of vitamin A to premature infants significantly reduced the incidence of BPD from 85% (17/20) in controls to 45% (9/20) in the treated group (Shenai et al., 1987). The use of supplemental vitamin A was also associated with a reduction in the need for respiratory aids or intensive care, and with a reduced incidence of airway infection and retinopathy of prematurity (Shenai et al., 1987).

C. Immune Function and Measles Morbidity

Vitamin A deficiency in animals is associated with pneumonia and infections, as well as a decreased resistance to pathogens. Vitamin A deficiency (in combination with general malnutrition) is also associated with increased risk of respiratory disease and diarrhea (Sommer et al., 1984) and increased mortality (Sommer et al., 1983; Sommer and West, 1987) in children. A deficiency of vitamin A is hypothesized to lower resistance to infection by preventing normal growth of mucus-secreting epithelial cells. Vitamin A may be important in other aspects of immune system protection; for example, in vitro, retinol significantly increases the tumor-killing activity of human monocytes (Moriguchi et al., 1988).

Treatment with supplemental vitamin A results in an increase in the normal antibody response to foreign proteins in laboratory animals (Cohen and Cohen, 1973; Nuwayri–Salti and Murad, 1985). However, vitamin A treatment (200,000 IU) did not enhance the antibody response to tetanus toxoid in young, malnourished Bangladeshi children (Brown et al., 1980). Nonetheless, semiannual treatment with that amount of vitamin A was associated with a significant reduction in mortality among Sumatran children (Tarwotjo et al., 1987). In an Australian study, apparently well–nourished children with a history of respiratory infections were randomized in a double–blind trial. Those who were supplemented with an average of 450 µg/day (1350 IU) of vitamin A for 11 months had 19% fewer episodes of respiratory symptoms than did subjects receiving a placebo (Pinnock et al., 1986). This difference was statistically significant.

Blindness and/or death due to measles are major problems among young children in developing countries in Africa and South Asia. Although malnutrition in general is associated with increased severity of measles (Dossetor et al., 1977), acute infections such as measles (Reddy et al., 1986; Varavithya et al., 1986) and chickenpox (Campos et al., 1987) will further depress vitamin A status. It has been hypothesized that the blindness and life–threatening diarrhea (which may appear some time after the attack of measles) result from depletion of marginal vitamin A stores by the disease (Laditan and Fafunso, 1981). Although significant morbidity is seen in poorly nourished children compromised by other diseases, the measles virus specifically affects epithelial cells, particularly mucous membranes of the lung and mouth, and so may put especially high demands on vitamin A stores. In fact, vitamin A status appears to be "critical" to the prognosis in cases of measles (*Lancet,* 1987). Inadequate vitamin A status in children with measles has been cited as a major cause of blindness in East Africa (Sauter, 1982). Children with measles were found to have lower serum vitamin A levels than healthy controls; children having both measles and early stages of eye damage had the lowest levels (Laditan and Fafunso, 1981). The eye involvement seen after a bout of measles responds to vitamin A supplementation (Reddy et al., 1986); however, there is some evidence that raising plasma retinol levels is not always effective in the treatment of postmeasles corneal lesions (James et al., 1984).

Vitamin A supplementation to marginally nourished children with measles (two 200,000 IU doses on consecutive days) was associated with a mortality rate of 7%, compared with 13% among unsupplemented patients (Barclay et al., 1987). In children under 2 years of age the difference in mortality was significant: 2.2% (1/46) among supplemented vs. 16.7% (7/42) among unsupplemented children. In May 1987 the World Health Organization and UNICEF issued a joint statement recommending treatment with vitamin A for "all children diagnosed with measles in communities in which vitamin A deficiency is a recognized problem" (WHO/UNICEF, 1987).

III. SAFETY

Acute hypervitaminosis A results from ingestion of very large amounts of the vitamin during a relatively short period of time. The symptoms, which resolve after supplementation is stopped, include irritability, headache, vomiting, bone pain, weakness, blurred vision, and peeling of the skin (Olson, 1984). Chronic hypervitaminosis A can result from high intakes of vitamin A over long periods of time and/or in connection with liver or kidney disease. Some of the signs of chronic hypervitaminosis A are dry skin, hair loss, weakness, headache, bone thickening, enlarged liver and spleen, anemia, abnormal menstrual periods, stiffness, and joint pain; most of these symptoms are reversible, but bone changes and liver damage may be permanent (Olson, 1984).

Vitamin A in very large doses is known to be teratogenic in many animals. Excessive intake of vitamin A has also been associated with human congenital abnormalities in some case reports, although a causal relationship has not been established (Bendich and Langseth 1989). High intakes (above the U.S. RDA of 8000 IU) should be avoided by pregnant women.

Levels of vitamin A intake associated with hypervitaminosis A vary according to the health and size of the person. As little as 12,000 IU/day, given to small children for an extended period, has reportedly led to toxicity symptoms (Bauernfeind, 1980). Hypervitaminosis A may result from acute ingestion of about 500,000 IU of vitamin A by an adult, or from a chronic daily intake of about 100,000 IU (Bendich and Langseth, 1989). The National Academy of Sciences Committee on Dietary Allowances stated that intake of more than 25,000 IU/day is "not prudent" (Committee on Dietary Allowances, 1980).

IV. SUMMARY

There is an association between low intake of carotene and vitamin A and increased risk of breast cancer. Low retinol intake is not consistently associated with an increased risk of developing lung, bladder, or prostate cancer. Vitamin A is effective in the treatment of some precancerous lesions, such as oral leukoplakia and esophageal dysplasia.

High-dose vitamin A supplementation to premature infants reduces morbidity and the incidence of bronchopulmonary dysplasia.

Poor vitamin A status is associated with compromised immune system function. Supplemental retinol may enhance immune function. The morbidity (particularly blindness) and mortality associated with measles infection in marginally nourished children can be reduced by high-dose supplementation with vitamin A.

Acute and chronic hypervitaminosis A cause potentially serious but generally reversible symptoms. Because very high doses of vitamin A are teratogenic in animals, pregnant women are cautioned against high–dose supplementation.

REFERENCES

Barclay, A. J. G., Foster, A., and Sommer, A. (1987). Vitamin A supplements and mortality related to measles: a randomised clinical trial. *Br. Med. J. 294*:294–296.

Bauernfeind, J. C. (1980). The safe use of vitamin A. A report of the International Vitamin A Consultative Groups (IVACC). The Nutrition Foundation, Washington, DC.

Bendich, A. and Langseth, L. (1989). Safety of vitamin A. *Am. J. Clin. Nutr. 49*:358–371.

Bond, G. G., Thompson, F. E., and Cook, R. R. (1987). Dietary vitamin A and lung cancer: results of a case-control study among chemical workers. *Nutr. Cancer 9*:109–121.

Brown, K. H., Rajan, M. M., Chakraborty, J., and Aziz, K. M. A. (1980). Failure of a large dose of vitamin A to enhance the antibody response to tetanus toxoid in children. *Am. J. Clin. Nutr. 33*:212–217.

Campos, F. A. C. S., Flores, H., and Underwood, B. A. (1987). Effect of an infection on vitamin A status of children as measured by the relative dose response (RDR). *Am. J. Clin. Nutr. 46*:91–94.

Cohen, B. E. and Cohen, I. K. (1973). Vitamin A: adjuvant and steroid antagonist in the immune response. *J. Immunol. 111*:1376–1380.

Committee on Dietary Allowances, Food and Nutrition Board (1980). *Recommended Dietary Allowances*, 9th rev. ed. National Academy of Sciences, Washington, DC.

Dossetor, J., Whittle, H. C., and Greenwood, B. M. (1977). Persistent measles infection in malnourished children. *Br. Med. J. 1*:1633–1635.

Friedman, G. D., Blaner, W. S., Goodman, D. S., Vogelman, J. H., Brind, J. L., Hoover, R., Fireman, B. H., and Orentreich, N. (1986). Serum retinol and retinol–binding protein levels do not predict subsequent lung cancer. *Am. J. Epidemiol. 123*:781–789.

Gregor, A., Lee, P. N., Roe, F. J. C., Wilson, M. J., and Melton, A. (1980). Comparison of dietary histories in lung cancer cases and controls with special reference to vitamin A. *Nutr. Cancer 2*:93–97.

Heshmat, M. Y., Kaul, L., Kovi, J., Jackson, M. A., Jackson, A. G., Jones, G. W., Edson, M., Enterline, J. P., Worrell, R. G., and Perry, S. L. (1985). Nutrition and prostate cancer: a case-control study. *Prostate 6*:7–17.

Humble, C. G., Samet, J. M., and Skipper, B. E. (1987). Use of quantified and frequency indices of vitamin A intake in a case-control study of lung cancer. *Int. J. Epidemiol. 16*:341–346.

Hustead, V. A., Gutcher, G. R., Anderson, S. A., and Zachman, R. D. (1984). Relationship of vitamin A (retinol) status to lung disease in the preterm infant. *J. Pediatr. 105*:610–615.

James, H. O., West, C. E., Duggan, M. B., and Ngwa, M. (1984). A controlled study on the effect of injected water-miscible retinyl palmitate on plasma concentrations of retinol and retinol-binding protein in children with measles in northern Nigeria. *Acta. Paediatr. Scand. 73*:22–28.

Kark, J. D., Smith, A. H., Switzer, B. R., and Hames, C. G. (1981). Serum vitamin A (retinol) and cancer incidence in Evans County, Georgia. *J. Natl. Cancer Inst. 66*:7–16.

Katsouyanni, K., Willett, W., Trichopoulos, D., Boyle, P., Trichopoulou, A., Vasilaros, S., Papadiamantis, J., and MacMahon, B. (1988). Risk of breast cancer among Greek women in relation to nutrient intake. *Cancer 61*:181–185.

Kaul, L., Heshmat, M. Y., Kovi, J., Jackson, M. A., Jackson, A. G., Jones, G. W., Edson, M., Enterline, J. P., Worrell, R. G., and Perry, S. L. (1987). The role of diet in prostate cancer. *Nutr. Cancer 9*:123–128.

Kolonel, L. N., Hankin, J. H., and Yoshizawa, C. N. (1987). Vitamin A and prostate cancer in elderly men: enhancement of risk. *Cancer Res. 47*:2982–2985.

Kummet, T., Moon, T. E., and Meyskens, F. L., Jr. (1983). Vitamin A: evidence for its preventive role in human cancer. *Nutr. Cancer 5*:96–106.

Laditan, A. A. O. and Fafunso, M. (1981). Serum levels of vitamin A, β-carotene and albumin in children with measles. *East Afr. Med. J. 58*:51–55.

Lancet Editorial (1987). Vitamin A for measles. *Lancet 1*:1067–1068.

Marubini, E., Decarli, A., Costa, A., Mazzoleni, C., Andreoli, C., Barbieri, A., Capitelli, E., Carlucci, M., Cavallo, F., Monferroni, N., Pastorino, U., and Salvini, S. (1988). The relationship of dietary intake and serum levels of retinol and β-carotene with breast cancer. *Cancer 61*:173–180.

Mehta, R. R., Hart, G., Beattie, C. W., and DasGupta, T. K. (1987). Significance of plasma retinol binding protein levels in recurrence of breast tumors in women. *Oncology 44*:350–355.

Mettlin, C., Selenskas, S., Natarajan, N., and Huben, R., (1989). Beta-carotene, animal fats and their relationship to prostate cancer risk: a case-control study. *Cancer 64*:605–612.

Michalek, A. M., Cummings, K. M., and Phelan, J. (1987). Vitamin A and tumor recurrence in bladder cancer. *Nutr. Cancer 9*:143–146.

Moriguchi, S., Werner, L., and Watson, R. R., (1985). High dietary vitamin A (retinyl palmitate) and cellular immune funtions in mice. *Immunol. 56*:169–177.

Moriguchi, S., Kohge, M., Kishino, Y., and Watson, R. R. (1988). In vitro effect of retinol and 13-*cis* retinoic acid on cytotoxicity of human monocytes. *Nutr. Res. 8*:255–264.

Nutrition Reviews (1986). Low plasma vitamin A levels in preterm neonates with bronchopulmonary dysplasia. *Nutr. Rev. 44*:202–204.

Nuwayri–Salti, N. and Murad, T. (1985). Immunologic and antiimmunosuppressive effects of vitamin A. *Pharmacology 30*:181–187.

Ohno, Y., Yoshida, O., Oishi, K., Okada, K., Yamabe, H., and Schroeder, F. H. (1988). Dietary β-carotene and cancer of the prostate: a case-control study in Kyoto, Japan. *Cancer Res. 48*:1331–1336.

Olson, J. A. (1984). Vitamin A. In *Handbook of Vitamins: Nutritional, Biochemical and Clinical Aspects*, L. J. Machlin, (Ed.). Marcel Dekker, New York, pp. 1–43.

Peleg, I., Heyden, S., Knowles, M., and Hames, C. G. (1984). Serum retinol and risk of subsequent cancer: extension of the Evans County, Georgia, study. *J. Natl. Cancer Inst. 73*:1455–1458.

Pinnock, C. B., Douglas, R. M., and Badcock, N. R. (1986). Vitamin A status in children who are prone to respiratory tract infections. *Aust. Paediatr. J. 22*:95–99.

Reddy, V., Bhaskaram, P., Raghuramulu, N., Milton, R. C., Rao, V., Madhusudan, J., and Radha Krishna, K. V. (1986). Relationship between measles, malnutrition, and blindness: a prospective study in Indian children. *Am. J. Clin. Nutr. 44*:24–30.

Rotkin, I. D., (1977). Studies in the epidemiology of prostatic cancer: expanded sampling. *Cancer Treat. Rep. 61*:173–180.

Samet, J. M., Skipper, B. J., Humble, C. G., and Pathak, D. R. (1985). Lung cancer risk and vitamin A consumption in New Mexico. *Am. Rev. Respir. Dis. 131*:198–202.

Sauter, J. J. M. (1982). Why measles makes so many children blind. *Trop. Doctor 12*:219–222.

Shenai J. P., Chytil, F., and Stahlman, M. T. (1985). Vitamin A status of neonates with bronchopulmonary dysplasia. *Pediatr. Res. 19*:185–188.

Shenai, J. P., Kennedy, K. A., Chytil, F., and Stahlman, M. T. (1987). Clinical trial of vitamin A supplementation in infants susceptible to bronchopulmonary dysplasia. *J. Pediatr. 111*:269–277.

Sommer, A. and West, K. P., Jr. (1987). Impact of vitamin A on childhood mortality. *Indian J. Pediatr. 54*:461–463.

Sommer, A., Hussaini, G., Tarwotjo, I., and Susanto, D. (1983). Increased mortality in children with mild vitamin A deficiency. *Lancet 2*:585–588.

Sommer, A., Katz, J., and Tarwotjo, I. (1984). Increased risk of respiratory disease and diarrhea in children with preexisting mild vitamin A deficiency. *Am. J. Clin. Nutr. 40*:1090–1095.

Sporn, M. B. and Roberts, A. B. (1983). Role of retinoids in differentiation and carcinogenesis. *Cancer Res. 43*:3034–3040.

Stich, H. F., Stich, W., Rosin, M. P., and Vallejera, M. O. (1984a). Use of the micronucleus test to monitor the effect of vitamin A, beta-carotene and canthaxanthin on the buccal mucosa of betel nut/tobacco chewers. *Int. J. Cancer 34*:745–750.

Stich, H. F., Rosin, M. P., and Vallejera, M. O. (1984b). Reduction with vitamin A and beta-carotene administration of proportion of micronucleated buccal mucosal cells in Asian betel nut and tobacco chewers. *Lancet 1*:1204–1206.

Stich, H. F., Hornby, A. P., Mathew, B., Sankaranarayanan, R., and Nair, M. K. (1988a). Response of oral leukoplakias to the administration of vitamin A. *Cancer Lett. 40*:93–101.

Stich, H. F., Rosin, M. P., Hornby, A. P., Mathew, B., Sankaranarayan an, R., and Nair, M. K. (1988b). Remission of oral leukoplakias and micronuclei in tobacco/betel quid chewers treated with beta-carotene and with beta-carotene plus vitamin A. *Int. J. Cancer 42*:195–199.

Tarwotjo, I., Sommer, A., West, K. P., Jr., Djunaedi, E., Mele, L., Hawkins, B., and the Aceh Study Group (1987). Influence of participation on mortality in a randomized trial of vitamin A prophylaxis. *Am. J. Clin. Nutr. 45*:1466–1471.

Tyler, H. A., Barr, L. C., Kissin, M. W., Westbury, G., and Dickerson, J. W. T. (1985). Vitamin A and non–epithelial tumours. *Br. J. Cancer* *51*:425–427.

Tyler, H. A, Notley, R. G., Schweitzer, F. A. W., and Dickerson, J. W. T. (1986). Vitamin A status and bladder cancer. *Eur. J. Surg. Oncol.* *12*:35–41.

Varavithya, W., Stoecker, B., Chaiyaratana, W., and Kittikool, J. (1986). Vitamin A status of Thai children with measles. *Trop. Geogr. Med.* *38*:359–361.

Wahi, P. N., Bodkhe, R. R., Arora, S., and Srivastava, M. C. (1962). Serum vitamin A studies in leukoplakia and carcinoma of the oral cavity. *Indian J. Pathol. Bact.* *5*:10–16.

Wahrendorf, J., Munoz, N., Jian–Bang, L., Thurnham, D. I., Crespi, M., and Bosch, F. X. (1988). Blood, retinol and zinc riboflavin [sic] status in relation to precancerous lesions of the esophagus: findings from a vitamin intervention trial in the People's Republic of China. *Cancer Res.* *48*:2280–2283.

Wald, N., Boreham, J., and Bailey, A. (1986). Serum retinol and subsequent risk of cancer. *Br. J. Cancer* *54*:957–961.

Wald, N., Idle, M., Boreham, J., and Bailey, A. (1980). Low serum–vitamin–A and subsequent risk of cancer: preliminary results of a prospective study. *Lancet*. *2*:813–815.

WHO/UNICEF Joint Statement, (1987). Vitamin A for measles. *Wkly. Epid.. Rec.* *19*:133–134.

Ziegler, R. G., Mason, T. J., Stemhagen, A., Hoover, R., Schoenberg, J. B., Gridley, G., Virgo, P. W., Altman, R., and Fraumeni, J. F., Jr. (1984). Dietary carotene and vitamin A and risk of lung cancer among white men in New Jersey. *J. Natl. Cancer Inst.* *73*:1429–1435.

3

β-Carotene

S. K. Gaby and V. N. Singh

I. INTRODUCTION

Carotenoids are a group of pigments that contribute to the yellow, orange, and/or red coloration of fruits and vegetables. Over 500 carotenoids have been identified in nature. β-carotene is the most plentiful in human foods and of greatest importance in terms of human nutrition.

Traditionally, β-carotene has been considered as a provitamin. However, several lines of evidence show that some of β-carotene's functions are independent of its provitamin A role. The nonvitamin A functions of β-carotene are based on its ability to quench singlet oxygen and to act as an antioxidant by scavenging free radicals. One of the well-established nonvitamin A uses of β-carotene, apparently related to its singlet oxygen quenching capacity, is in the treatment of patients with erythropoietic protoporphyria (EPP), an inherited light-sensitive skin disorder. In addition, antioxidant and antimutagenic properties of this nutrient are thought to play roles in reducing the risk of certain types of cancer.

II. ANTIOXIDANT AND SINGLET OXYGEN QUENCHING PROPERTIES

A. Singlet Oxygen Quencher

β-Carotene is the most effective naturally occurring quencher of singlet oxygen, a reactive, highly energized molecule (Foote et al., 1970). Due to its instability and high energy level, singlet oxygen can potentially pass along this energy to other molecules. In the process, unstable chemical species (free radicals) can be generated.

Specific structural features of β-carotene enable it to quench singlet oxygen and prevent the generation of free radicals (and the damage they cause). β-carotene is a long molecule held together by 11 conjugated double bonds, i.e., double bonds alternating between single chemical bonds. As β-carotene is relatively large, it can distribute energy over all of its double and single bonds. The energy transferred to β-carotene can be released as heat, restoring β-carotene to its original energy level. This reaction does not destroy the β-carotene molecule but transforms singlet oxygen into a stable oxygen species lacking the energy to engage in harmful reactions. It has been calculated that one molecule of β-carotene can quench up to 1000 molecules of singlet oxygen (Foote et al., 1970). Other carotenoids having a minimum of nine conjugated double bonds also have the ability to quench singlet oxygen (Foote et al., 1970). Canthaxanthin, a carotenoid closely resembling β-carotene, exhibits singlet oxygen quenching properties but has no provitamin A activity.

B. Antioxidant Function

In addition to preventing free radical formation resulting from reactions involving singlet oxygen, β-carotene can react with or scavenge free radicals directly and thus act as an antioxidant.

The mechanism by which β-carotene halts this damaging process has been examined by Burton and Ingold (1984), who found that β-carotene is a chain-breaking antioxidant. Unlike antioxidants that prevent the initiation of lipid peroxidation, β-carotene stops the chain reaction by trapping free radicals. According to Burton and Ingold, β-carotene is an unusual type of lipid antioxidant in that it is most effective at the low oxygen concentrations found in capillary beds in tissues far removed from direct exposure to oxygen (1984). The antioxidant function of β-carotene might complement the action of other antioxidant protective molecules, such as catalase, glutathione peroxidase, vitamin C, and vitamin E, which are not as effective at lower oxygen concentrations. Vitamin A, in contrast, is a very weak antioxidant and does not quench singlet oxygen.

III. HEALTH BENEFITS

A. Photoprotection

The process of photosynthesis produces large amounts of free radicals. Plants are protected from the lethal oxidation caused by photosynthesis by antioxidant pigments such as β-carotene (Schrott, 1985). Photosynthetic bacteria also synthesize carotenoids to prevent free radical damage (Sistrom et al., 1956). When mutant blue-green bacteria that had lost their natural pigments were exposed to air and light, 98% were killed and many of the survivors were damaged (Sistrom et al., 1956). By contrast, the non-mutated bacteria containing carotenoids grew normally when exposed to light and air.

Observations of the photoprotective effect of carotenoids in a wide variety of living systems (Sistrom et al., 1956) led to the use of β-carotene in the successful treatment of patients with inherited light-sensitive skin disorders (Table B1) (see Mathews–Roth, 1986, for review).

Erythropoietic protoporphyria is an inherited light-sensitive disease. This disease is characterized by burning, redness, and swelling of skin when exposed to the sun. In a large 7-year study designed by Mathews-Roth, the effectiveness of β-carotene supplementation was examined in 133 patients with EPP. The results indicated that 84% of the patients increased their ability to tolerate sunlight exposure without development of symptoms (Mathews-Roth et al., 1970, 1974). Since these original studies, many other patients have shown an increased tolerance to sunlight when treated with β-carotene (Mathews-Roth et al., 1977; Thomsen et al., 1979).

This treatment often requires the use of β-carotene in high doses (up to 180 mg/day). No serious side effects from β-carotene ingestion have been reported.

The success of β-carotene therapy in patients with EPP has resulted in attempts to use β-carotene for other light sensitive skin disorders. β-carotene may be of some value in patients with congenital porphyria (Sneddon, 1974; Baart de la Faille and Remme, 1979).

B. Immunoenhancement

Recent findings indicate that carotenoids can enhance some aspects of immune function. This immunoenhancement is also seen with carotenoids that lack provitamin A activity.

Several animal studies have shown that there is improved immune function following supplementation with β-carotene (Bendich and Shapiro, 1986; Schwartz et al., 1986; Schwartz and Shklar, 1987; Tomita et al., 1987), including improved tumor resistance (Seifter et al., 1983, 1984; Schwartz and Shklar, 1988). β-carotene has been shown to enhance both specific and nonspecific immune responses in experimental animals and in vitro models (Bendich, 1988a).

Immune system response to short–term, high–dose β-carotene supplementation was examined in one human trial. Supplements of 180 mg

Table 1. Effects of Carotenoids on Human Light Sensitive Skin Disorders

Skin disorders	Effect	Reference
Erythropoietic protoporphyria	87% of patients with EPP increased their ability to tolerate sunlight when treated with oral β–carotene(15–180 mg/day)	Mathews-Roth et al. (1974)
Erythropoietic protoporphyria	Of 36 patients treated with β–carotenealone or β–carotene+ canthaxanthin(50–100 mg/day) 100% experienced improvement in their condition	Thomsen et al. (1979)
Congential porphyria	18-year-old patient treated with 25 mg β–carotene/day was found to tolerate sunlight without suffering blister formation	Sneddon (1974)
Congenital porphyria	Daily doses of β–carotene/canthaxanthin (150 mg) increased tolerance to sunlight in a female patient	Baart de la Faille and Remme (1979)
Polymorphous light eruption	33% of patients treated with oral β–carotene (15–180 mg/day) showed improved tolerance to sunlight	Mathews-Roth et al. (1977)
Polymorphous light eruption	β–carotene (30–300 mg/day) increased photoprotection in 72% of patients	Fusaro and Johnson (1980)
Polymorphous light eruption	6/19 of patients receiving 3mg/kg body weight β–carotene experienced complete remission	Parrish et al.(1979)
Actinic reticuloid, solar urticaria	No evidence of improvement in 5 patients receiving 15–150 mg/day despite high serum carotene levels	Kobza et al. (1973)
Solar urticaria, hydroa aestivale, actinic reticuloid, or porphyria cutanea tarda	One-fifth of patients increased their protection index when treated with β–carotene	Mathews-Roth et al. (1977)

β-carotene per day for 2 weeks increased the number of T_4 lymphocytes (helper cells) and did not effect T_8 lymphocytes (suppressor cells) (Alexander et al., 1985).

C. Cancer

1. Cancer Risk and Dietary Intake or Blood Level of β-Carotene/Carotenoids

More than 50 epidemiological studies conducted during the last decade in different parts of the world have consistently demonstrated that a high intake of foods rich in β-carotene is associated with reduced risk of certain cancers, especially lung cancer (Tables 2, 3, and 4). Increased β-carotene consumption has also been found to be associated with reduced risk of cancers of the cervix, esophagus, and stomach, although these findings are not as overwhelming as in the case of lung cancer.

2. Lung Cancer

A sizable number of studies on β-carotene intake and serum levels have shown an association between high β-carotene intake and/or status and reduced risk of lung cancer (Table 2).

The studies of diet and lung cancer show a remarkably consistent protective effect of β-carotene from green and yellow fruits and vegetables. In more than 25 different studies groups of individuals with the highest consumption of these foods (or having the highest blood levels of β-carotene) generally had half the risk of developing this cancer than those with the lowest intake or blood levels of β-carotene had (MacLennan et al., 1977; Hirayama, 1979; Mettlin et al., 1979; Shekelle et al., 1981; Graham 1983; Kvale et al., 1983; Hinds et al., 1984; Nomura et al., 1985; Samet et al., 1985; Wu et al., 1985; Menkes et al., 1986; Pisani et al., 1986; Ziegler et al., 1986; Bond et al., 1987; Byers et al., 1987; Gey et al., 1987; Humble et al., 1987; Pastorino et al., 1987; Koo 1988; Wald et al., 1988; Connett et al., 1989; Kune et al., 1989; LeMarchand et al., 1989; Mettlin, 1989).

A large prospective dietary study (data collection before cancer diagnosis), by Shekelle et al., followed 1954 men employed by Western Electric Co., Chicago, for 19 years (1981). This study was important since it differentiated between a "carotene index" based on consumption of fruits and vegetables and a "retinol index" based on intake of preformed retinol from animal sources. There was a sevenfold increase in the risk of lung cancer in smokers whose carotene index fell in the lowest quartile, as compared to those in the highest quartile of intake. The intake of retinol rich foods was not related to the risk of lung cancer.

Table 2.   Epidemiological Studies of β-Carotene and Lung Cancer

Study	Parameter measured[a]	Outcome[b]
Bjelke, 1975	Total dietary vitamin A (P)	+
Maclennan et al., 1977	Dark-green leafy vegetables (R)	+
Hirayama, 1979	Green/yellow vegetables (P)	+
Mettlin et al., 1979	Carrots (R)	+
Gregor et al., 1980	Total dietary vitamin A (R)	+
Shekelle et al., 1981	Dietary carotene (P)	+
Kvale et al., 1983	Carrots (P)	+
Hinds et al., 1984	Dietary carotene (R)	+
Willett et al., 1984	Serum carotenes (P)	0
Samet et al., 1985	Dietary carotene (R)	+
Wu et al., 1985	Dietary β-carotene (R)	+
Nomura et al., 1985	Serum β-carotene (P)	+
Menkes et al., 1986	Serum β-carotene (P)	+
Pisani et al., 1986	Carrots (R)	+
Ziegler et al., 1986	Dark-yellow/orange vegetables (R)	+
Bond et al., 1987	Plant foods (R)	+
Byers et al., 1987	Fruits and vegetables (R)	+
Gey et al., 1987	Serum β-carotene (P)	+
Humble et al., 1987	Dietary carotene (R)	+
Kromhout, 1987	Dietary β-carotene (P)	0
Paganini-Hill et al., 1987	Dietary β-carotene (P)	0
Pastorino et al., 1987	Dietary β-carotene (R)	+
Fontham et al., 1988	Dietary carotene (R)	+
Holst et al., 1988	Dietary β-carotene (R)	0
Koo, 1988	Carrots and green leafy vegetables (R)	+
Wald et al., 1988	Serum β-carotene (P)	+
Kune et al., 1989	Serum β-carotene (R)	+
Mettlin, 1989	Dietary β-carotene (R)	+
LeMarchand et al., 1989	Dietary β-carotene (R)	+
Connet et al., 1989	Serum β-carotene (P)	+

[a]Letter in parentheses indicates study type.   R = retrospective;   P = prospective.
[b] + = association found between high intake/status and reduced cancer risk. 0 = no association found between intake/status and cancer risk.

Menkes and colleagues (1986) found significantly lower levels of serum β-carotene among 99 persons who later developed lung cancer as compared with controls. Moreover, the risk of cancer increased as serum levels of β-carotene decreased. This association between low levels of serum β-carotene and increased risk of lung cancer was also described in three other studies (Nomura et al., 1985; Gey et al., 1987; Wald et al.,1988; Connett et al., 1989). Individuals known to have lung cancer have also been reported to have significantly lower serum β-carotene levels than controls (Pastorino et al., 1987).

There were four studies in which carotenoid intake or plasma carotene status was not associated with decreased lung cancer risk. In one study (Willett et al., 1984) the participants were all taking medications for cardiovascular disease and total serum carotenoids, not β-carotene, were measured. [The use of certain medicines may represent a significant confounder in this study. It was reported in a recent large study that the use of anti-hypertensive drugs was associated with reduced plasma β-carotene levels (Nierenberg et al., 1989).] A large prospective study of diet found that β -carotene tended to have an inverse relationship with 25–year lung cancer mortality, however, this trend was not statistically significant (Kromhout 1987). Holst et al.(1988) did not find a protective effect of β-carotene intake in small case–control study. In that trial all types of lung cancer are considered together, and fewer than a third were squamous cell carcinoma (SCC). This may render inconclusive any findings on a β-carotene effect, which appears to be most protective against SCC of the lung (Ziegler et al.,1986). In another study where no protective effect of β-carotene was found, all participants had very high total vitamin A intakes (Paganini–Hill et al., 1987).

Carotene Status of Cigarette Smokers   Many studies have found lower levels of carotene/β-carotene in smokers (Witter et al., 1982; Russell-Briefel et al., 1985; Davis et al., 1983; Chow et al., 1986; Stryker et al., 1987). Smokers ingesting the same amount of β-carotene as nonsmokers achieve lower serum levels of β-carotene (Stryker et al., 1988), suggesting that the smokers have altered metabolism of and greater need for the nutrient. Smokers are approximately 15 times more likely to develop lung cancer than nonsmokers (Byers et al., 1987).

3.   Cervical and Endometrial Cancer

High dietary intake and high serum levels of β-carotene have been associated with reduced risk of cervical and endometrial cancer (Table 3).

In a case-control study, decreased risk of severe cervical dysplasia or in situ carcinoma was associated with a dietary β-carotene intake above the median (Wylie-Rosett et al., 1984). Other studies also found strong associations between decreased risk of cervical cancer and high dietary intake of β-carotene (LaVecchia et al., 1984) and total carotene (Verreault et al., 1989). However, a negative association between invasive cervical cancer risk and total dietary carotene did not remain significant when adjusted for other risk factors (Verreault et al.,1989). Marshall et al., (1983) reported a decreased risk for cervical cancer with a high intake of fruits and vegetables, notably carrots and broccoli, rich in provitamin A carotenoids .

In a study assessing carotene consumption in 206 cases of endometrial cancer and 206 controls, high intake was associated with half the risk of developing the cancer compared to the low intake group (LaVecchia et al., 1986).

Orr et al., (1985) showed that serum β-carotene levels when examined prospectively were lower in patients who developed cervical and endometrial cancer. No difference in serum retinol levels in women with or without cancer was found. Harris et al., (1986) found a trend toward low serum β-carotene in cases of preinvasive disease of the cervix, although there was no relationship to invasive cancer. In a case–control study, women with plasma β-carotene levels in the highest quartile had an 80% reduction in risk of in situ cervical cancer, after adjusting for established risk factors for cervical cancer, in comparison with those whose levels were in the lowest quartile (Brock et al., 1988). In another report plasma levels of β-carotene were significantly lower in women with mild cervical dysplasia than in controls; still lower levels were associated with severe dysplasia or in situ carcinoma, and the lowest levels were reported in

Table 3.   Epidemiological Studies of β-Carotene and Gynecological Cancers

Study	Parameter measured[a]	Outcome[b]
	Breast	
Wald et al., 1984	Serum β-carotene (P)	+
Willett et al., 1984	Serum carotenes (P)	0
LaVecchia et al., 1987a	Dietary β-carotene (R)	+
Katsouyanni et al., 1988	Dietary carotene (R)	+
Rohan et al., 1988	Dietary β-carotene (R)	+
Marubini et al., 1988	Diet and serum β-carotene (R)	0
	Cervix	
Marshall et al., 1983	Dietary β-carotene (R)	+
LaVecchia et al., 1984	Dietary β-carotene (R)	+
Wylie-Rosett et al., 1984	Dietary β-carotene (R)	+
Brock et al., 1988	Dietary β-carotene (R)	+
Verreault et al., 1989	Dietary carotene (R)	0
	Cervix/endometrium	
Hirayama, 1979	Green/yellow vegetables (P)	+
Orr et al., 1985	Serum β-carotene (P)	+
LaVecchia et al., 1986	Dietary β-carotene (R)	+

[a]Letter in parentheses indicates study type.   R = retrospective;   P = prospective.
[b] + = association found between high intake/status and reduced cancer risk. 0 = no association found between intake/status and cancer risk.

cancer cases (Palan et al., 1988). There were no significant differences in plasma retinol levels (Fig. 1).

4. Esophageal Cancer

Dietary β-carotene has been inversely associated with esophageal cancer risk (Table 4).

Relatively high intake of β-carotene-rich foods (vegetables and fruit) was associated with a lower risk of death from esophageal cancer in a case-control, retrospective study of black males (Ziegler et al., 1981). However, the population studied had a generally poor diet and the data may represent differences between malnourished and less poorly nourished groups. In a comparatively well-nourished group in France, in an area with a high incidence of esophageal cancer, a case-control study of diet showed a decreased relative risk of esophageal cancer associated with an increased carotene consumption (Tuyns et al., 1987).

Decarli and others (1987) found an association between the incidence of esophageal cancer and the frequency of consumption of carrots, green vegetables, and fresh fruit. The group with the highest carotene intake had one-fourth the risk of developing this cancer, compared with the group with the lowest intake. Another case-control study found a negative association between reduced esophageal cancer risk and total fruit consumption, but no association between risk and an index of dietary carotene (Brown et al., 1988).

5. Stomach Cancer

Decreased risk of stomach cancer has been associated with increased fruit and/or vegetable intake (Table 4). A study in China found low vegetable intake to be a risk factor for gastric cancer (Hu et al., 1988). Low fruit intake was associated with increased risk in a study in Japan (Kono et al.,1988), where the incidence of gastric cancer is extremely high. Decreased stomach cancer risk was also associated with frequent green vegetable consumption (LaVecchia et al., 1987b), daily green and yellow vegetable consumption (Hirayama, 1979), and high intakes of selected carotene—containing fruits and vegetables (but not total carotenes) (Modan et al., 1981).

Blood levels of β-carotene were found to be significantly lower in individuals with gastric dysplasia (Haenszel et al., 1985), a precancerous condition. Reduced serum levels of β-carotene were associated with increased risk in a prospective study of gastric cancer (Gey et al., 1987). In a recent study, low serum β-carotene was associated with an increased risk of developing stomach cancer, although the number of cases was small (Wald et

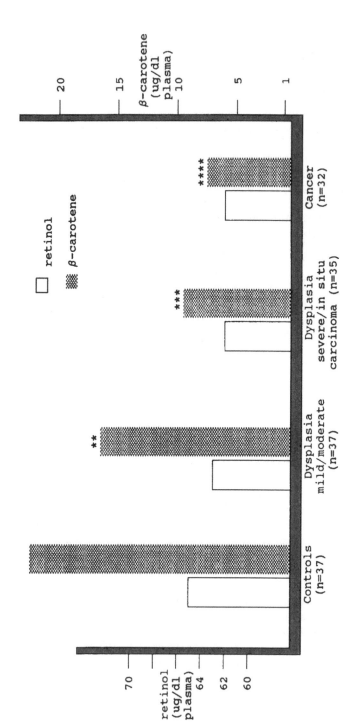

Figure 1. Mean plasma retinol and β-carotene levels in control subjects and women with cervical dysplasia and squamous cell carcinoma of the cervix (Palan et al., 1988). **Controls vs. mild dysplasia, *P*<0.001;*** mild vs. severe, *P*<0.001;**** severe vs. cancer, *P*<0.05.

Table 4.   Epidemiological Studies of β-Carotene and Gastrointestinal Cancers

Study	Parameter measured[a]	Outcome[b]
	Esophagus	
Cook-Mozaffari et al., 1979	Fresh fruit and vegetables (R)	+
Ziegler et al., 1981	Dietary carotene (R)	+
Decarli et al., 1987	Dietary β-carotene (R)	+
Tuyns et al., 1987	Dietary carotene (R)	+
Hirayama, 1979	Green/yellow vegetables (P)	+
Brown et al., 1988	Fruit/carotene (R)	+/0
	Stomach	
Wynder et al., 1963	Fruit and vegetables (R)	+
Hirayama, 1979	Green/yellow vegetables (P)	+
Gey et al., 1987	Serum β-carotene (P)	+
LaVecchia et al., 1987b	Green vegetables (R)	+
Hu et al., 1988	Vegetables (R)	+
You et al., 1988	Fresh fruit and vegetables (R)	+
Wald et al., 1988	Serum β-carotene (P)	+
Kono et al., 1988	Fruit (R)	+
Buiatti et al., 1989	Fruit and raw vegetables (R)	+
	Gastrointestinal Tract	
Modan et al., 1981	Carotene-containing	+
	Fruits and vegetables (R)	
Willett et al., 1984	Serum carotenes (P)	0
	Colon	
Phillips, 1975	Green leafy vegetables (R)	0
Hirayama, 1979	Green/yellow vegetables (P)	+
Tomkin et al., 1986	Total dietary vitamin A (R)	0
Kune and Kune, 1987	Fruits and vegetables (R)	0
Young and Wolf, 1988	Vegetables (R)	+
Slattery et al., 1988	Fruit and vegetables (R)	+
West et al., 1989	Dietary β-carotene (R)	+
	Colon/rectum	
Shekelle et al., 1981	Dietary carotene (P)	0
Gey et al., 1987	Plasma β-carotene (P)	0
Wu et al., 1987	Dietary β-carotene (P)	0
LaVecchia et al., 1988	Green vegetables (R)	+

[a]R = retrospective study;   P = prospective study.
[b] + = Association found between high intake/status and reduced cancer risk. 0 = no association found between intake/status and cancer risk.

al., 1988). *Total* serum carotenoids were not related to gastric cancer risk in another trial (Willett et al., 1984).

6. Breast Cancer

High serum level and/or dietary intake of carotene/β-carotene has been associated with lowered risk of developing breast cancer in four studies; one study found no association (Marubini et al., 1988). Both carotenes and retinol were found to contribute to the moderately decreased risk for developing breast cancer (Katsouyanni et al., 1988). Also, more frequent green vegetable consumption was associated with decreased risk of breast cancer (LaVecchia et al., 1987a). A recent study found a statistically significant trend toward decreasing risk of breast cancer associated with increasing β-carotene intake (but not retinol intake) (Rohan et al., 1988).

In a study by Wald et al., (1984) serum β-carotene levels tended to be lower in 39 women who later developed breast cancer than in 78 women who did not develop breast cancer (Table 3).

Increased carotenoid (but not retinol) intake was associated with a reduction in tissue densities, which are associated with increased breast cancer risk (Brisson et al., 1989). These preliminary findings are intriguing and begin to address the problem of elucidating the mechanism by which β-carotene may reduce breast cancer risk.

7. Oral Precancer and Cancer

Snuff contains mutagenic substances. People who chew excessive amounts of snuff frequently exhibit precancerous and cancerous lesions in the mouth. The presence of micronucleated cells (MNC) at the site in the mouth where the tobacco is usually kept is used as an indicator of the chromosomal damage induced by tobacco .

Following β-carotene supplementation, an increase in the β-carotene concentration in oral mucosal cells in most subjects (Stitch et al.,1986) was accompanied by lower numbers of MNC (Stitch et al.,1984).

Members of the Ifugao tribe in the Philippines use snuff. Ifugaos who received B-carotene (180 mg/week) for 9 weeks had 66% fewer MNC than those who did not receive the β-carotene. Vitamin A treatment also significantly lowered the incidence of MNC. Canthaxanthin, a carotenoid which cannot be converted to vitamin A by humans, was ineffective. The effectiveness of the vitamin A treatment may have been due to improvement of the vitamin A status of these individuals. Vitamin A is essential for maintenance of the epithelial lining of the mouth. β-carotene may have served as a source of vitamin A as well as a free radical quencher (Stitch et al.,1984).

A second study with Inuits from the Northwest Territories of Canada, who also chew tobacco and have precancerous oral lesions, demonstrated that β-carotene may have antimutagenic properties independent of its provitamin A activity. Unlike the Ifugaos, the Inuits have a normal vitamin A status. In this study the group who received β-carotene (180 mg/week) for 10 weeks had 70% fewer MNC than the group that did not receive β-carotene (Stitch et al.,1985). Since both groups were vitamin A sufficient, the effectiveness of β-carotene in this population is unlikely to be solely due to its conversion to vitamin A.

A study in India demonstrated lower serum vitamin A and carotene levels in patients with oral leukoplakia (a precancerous condition) than in controls (Wahi et al.,1962). Similar results were reported in another study of oral cancer (Clifford 1972). However, both groups studied had a very poor nutritional status, especially with respect to both carotene and vitamin A. In several studies in western populations, where the vitamin A status is unlikely to be poor, serum carotene levels were lower in oral cancer patients than in controls (Abels et al., 1941; Basu et al.,1974; Autokorala et al.,1979; Harris et al.,1986; Pastorino et al.1987; Brock et al.; 1988).

Another recent study conducted in India showed a reduction in MNC, inhibition of oral leukoplakias, and remission of existing leukoplakias in tobacco/betel quid chewers supplemented with β-carotene (180 mg/week) (Stitch et al., 1988). Garewal et al., (1989) found that 82% of subjects had a significant favorable response to β-carotene supplementation (30 mg/day x 6 months) in a preliminary study of oral leukoplakia in a U.S. population.

8. All Cancers

A relationship was found between dietary intake of carotene from vegetables and subsequent 5 year mortality from cancer in 1271 residents of Massachusetts, 66 years of age or older (Colditz et al., 1985). After controlling for age and smoking behavior, those with the highest intake of carotene–containing vegetables had a threefold lower risk of cancer mortality than those with the lowest intake.

A large prospective study conducted in England showed an association between serum β-carotene levels and subsequent cancer incidence (Wald et al., 1988). The mean β-carotene levels of subjects who developed any type of cancer were significantly lower than the levels of matched controls. The association was strongest for cancers of the lung and stomach.

9. Limitations of Epidemiological Studies

Epidemiological studies have some inherent limitations. Prospective studies are generally quite reliable, but prolonged storage and repeated thaw-

ing of the samples before analysis may destroy nutrients and may therefore lead to an underestimation of their levels. Retrospective studies have
other limitations. It is difficult to differentiate between cause and effect
because data are collected when the disease has already developed. Additionally, the accuracy of food consumption data may be doubtful.

Some studies report associations with certain foods rather than β-carotene. In addition, very few foods have been analyzed for the various types
of carotenoids, so that even when β-carotene is considered separately, it is
usually estimated.

However, measurement of serum β-carotene levels (a good indicator of
consumption) can allow a more specific association between the nutrient
and cancer risk than can dietary recall. Indeed, serum analysis has shown
an association between high serum β-carotene levels and reduced risk of
certain cancers. It may also be the case that plasma carotenes are a
marker for the intake of certain fruits and vegetables, which have numerous beneficial components.

Despite the limitations, the large number of studies and the consistency
of the findings provide compelling evidence in support of β-carotene's role
in reducing the risk of certain types of cancer, particularly lung cancer.

10. Summary of Epidemiological Evidence

Results of epidemiological studies examining the association between
carotene/β-carotene intake and the incidence of certain cancers are summarized in Tables 2, 3 and 4. The most significant pattern that emerges is
that β-carotene seems to be most protective against lung cancer. A strong
association between low levels of carotene and greater cancer risk has been
reported for cancer of the cervix, esophagus, gastrointestinal tract, lung,
oropharynx/head and neck, and stomach. The majority of cancers at these
sites are of the epithelial cell type.

No protective effect has been consistently associated with intake of vitamin A and cancer of the cervix, esophagus, or lung. These findings suggest
that β-carotene may have specific protective effects at these cancer sites
independent of its provitamin A activity.

11. Possible Mechanisms for β-Carotene Anti–cancer Activity

The hypothesis that it is the β-carotene in the high β-carotene foods analyzed in epidemiological studies which provides the apparent
chemopreventive action is supported by strong scientific rationale and animal experiments.

β-carotene may be protective against cancer through its antioxidant
function, since oxidative products can cause genetic damage. Also, the

photoprotective properties of β-carotene may protect against UV–light–induced carcinogenesis.

Immunoenhancement by β-carotene, which may contribute to cancer protection, has been demonstrated in animal models. For example, tumor immunity was stimulated in a dose–dependent manner in mice fed β-carotene (Tomita et al., 1987).

Experiments with animals have shown that high-dose supplemental β-carotene protects against UV-light- and chemically-induced cancers, blocks cancer progression, stimulates immune responses, and is antitcarcinogenic (Santamaria et al., 1988). β-carotene may also have an anti-carcinogenic effect by altering liver metabolism of carcinogens (Basu et al., 1987).

12.   β-Carotene, Carotenoids, or Vitamin A?

Multivariate analyses can distinguish between the effects of carotenes (plant sources of vitamin A) and retinol (animal sources of vitamin A). A consistent pattern of a lack of association between intake of preformed vitamin A and cancer incidence and a significant association between high intake of carotene-rich foods and lower incidence of certain cancers has been seen in seventeen studies (Ziegler et al., 1981 and 1986; Winn et al., 1984; Samet et al., 1985; Wu et al., 1985; Pisani et al., 1986; LaVecchia et al., 1986, 1987a and b, and 1988a; Byers et al., 1987; Decarli et al., 1987; Humble et al., 1987; Pastorino et al., 1987; Tuyns et al., 1987; Brock et al., 1988; Rohan et al., 1988) (Tables 5 and 6). In addition, studies have shown a lack of association between serum retinol level and cancer risk, and an association between serum β-carotene level and cancer risk, yet a significant association between high serum β-carotene and reduced cancer risk (Table 7). It should be noted, however, that serum retinol level is generally a poor indicator of vitamin A status, except in cases of deficiency.

The epidemiological data do not provide clear evidence to differentiate the effects of β-carotene from those of other carotenoids. Nevertheless, Ziegler et al., (1986) showed that foods particularly rich in β-carotene, dark orange–yellow vegetables, were more strongly associated with reduced risk of lung cancer than vegetables and fruits rich in other carotenoids. Based on these findings, they concluded that β-carotene is probably responsible for the protective effect. In addition, some studies have shown a cancer risk reduction associated specifically with carrots (Mettlin et al., 1979; LaVecchia et al., 1984; Norell et al., 1986; Pisani et al., 1986; Bond et al., 1987; Decarli et al., 1987; Koo 1988; LaVecchia et al., 1989); carrots contain large amounts of β-carotene but very little of any of the other carotenoids. Also, the single prospective study of serum carotenoids that did not show an association between high levels and reduced cancer risk meas-

Table 5. Dietary Carotenes vs. Vitamin A: Risk of Cancers (Other Than Lung Cancer)—Retrospective Studies

| Site | Association with cancer risk | | Reference |
	Carotene	Vitamin A	
Bladder	+ (vegetables)	+ (milk)	Graham, 1983
Bladder	+ (carotenoids)	0 (retinoids)	LaVecchia et al., 1989
Breast	+ (carotenes)	+ (retinol)	Katsouyanni et al., 1988
Breast	+ (β-carotene)	0 (retinol)	LaVecchia et al., 1987a
Breast	+ (β-carotene)	0 (retinol)	Rohan et al., 1988
Colon	0 (carotene)	+ (retinol)	Tomkin et al., 1986
Cervix	+ (β-carotene)	0 (retinol)	Brock et al., 1988
Cervix	+ (β-carotene)	0 (retinol)	LaVecchia et al., 1988a
Endometrium	+ (β-carotene)	0 (retinol)	LaVecchia et al., 1986
Esophagus	+ (carotene)	0 (dairy/eggs)	Ziegler et al., 1981
Esophagus	+ (β-carotene)	0 (retinol)	Decarli et al., 1987
Esophagus	+ (β-carotene)	0 (retinol)[a]	Tuyns et al., 1987
Larynx	+ (carotene)	0 (retinol)	Mackerras et al., 1988
Oropharynx/ head and neck	+ (fruits and vegetables)	0 (dairy/eggs)	Winn et al., 1984
Stomach	+ (green vegetables)	0 (retinol)	LaVecchia et al., 1987b
Stomach	+ (carotene)	0 (retinol)	You et al., 1988

+ = increased risk of cancer with lower intake of carotene (particularly β-carotene) or vitamin A-containing foods.
0 = no association between the risk of cancer and a lower intake of carotene or vitamin A-containing foods.
[a]Retinol from butter and offal was associated with an increased risk with higher intake; retinol from other foods (e.g., eggs and milk) was not associated with an increased risk.

Table 6. Dietary Carotenes vs. Vitamin A: Lung Cancer Risk—Retrospective
Studies

Association with cancer risk		
Carotene	Vitamin A	Reference
+ (carrots)	+ (milk)	Mettlin et al., 1979
+ (carotene)	0 (retinol)	Shekelle et al., 1981
+ (vegetables)	+ (milk)	Kvale et al., 1983
+ (carotene)	0 (preformed)	Samet et al., 1985
+ (fruits and vegetables)	0 (retinol)	Byers et al., 1987
+ (carotene)	0 (retinol)	Ziegler et al., 1986
+ (carotene)	0 (preformed)	Wu et al., 1985
+ (carrots)	0 (liver/cheese)	Pisani et al., 1986
+ (plant foods)	+ (total vitamin A[a])	Bond et al., 1987
+ (carotene)	0 (retinol)	Humble et al., 1987
0 (β-carotene)	0 (total vitamin A[a])	Paganini-Hill et al., 1987
+ (β-carotene)	0 (retinol)	Pastorino et al., 1987
+ (carrots and green leafy vegetables)	+ (retinol)	Koo, 1988

+ = increased risk of cancer with lower intake of carotene (particularly β-carotene) or vitamin A-containing foods.
0 = no association between the risk of cancer and a lower intake of carotene or vitamin
A-containing foods.
[a]Total dietary vitamin A, including β-carotene.

ured total carotenoids (Willett et al., 1984); the studies that measured
β-carotene specifically found an association between β-carotene status and
cancer risk (Wald et al., 1984; Orr et al., 1985; Haenszel et al., 1985;
Nomura et al., 1985; Menkes et al., 1986; Gey et al., 1987).

Based on the above studies, it is reasonable to conclude that the observed reduction in cancer risk associated with certain foods is most likely
due to β-carotene. It may be valuable in the future to consider a dietary
recommendation for β-carotene separate from the vitamin A recommendation.

D. Cataracts

The changes in the structure of the lens of the eye which result in the formation of a cataract have been linked to oxidative stress and free radical
damage (Varma et al., 1984). The eye is exposed to a great deal of ultravio-

Table 7.   Serum Levels of Carotenes vs. Vitamin A: Cancer Risk

| Site | Association with cancer risk | | Study type[c] | Reference |
	β–Carotene[a]	Vitamin A[b]		
Breast	+	0	P	Wald et al., 1984
Breast	0 (carotene)	0	P	Willett et al., 1984
Cervix/endo-metrium	+	0	P	Orr et al., 1985
Cervix uteri	+	0	R	Harris et al., 1986
Cervix	+	0	R	Brock et al., 1988
Gastrointes-tinal tract	0 (carotene)	+	P	Willett et al., 1984
Lung	+	0	P	Gey et al., 1987
Lung	+	0	P	Nomura et al., 1985
Lung	+	0	P	Menkes et al., 1986
Lung	0 (carotene)	0	P	Willet et al., 1984
Stomach[d]	+	0	P	Haenszel et al,. 1985
Stomach	+	+	P	Gey et al., 1987

+ = increased risk of cancer with lower serum level of β-carotene or vitamin A.

0 = no association between risk of cancer and a lower serum level of β-carotene or vitamin A.

[a]β-Carotene serum fraction specifically measured except where indicated by carotene.
[b]Retinol serum levels measured.
[c]R = Retrospective, P = Prospective

[d]Low β-carotene levels associated with precancerous gastric dysplasia; subsequent cancer development was not reported.

let light, and cataract occurs most frequently in the elderly (in whom there has been long-term exposure to oxidation damage).

The appearance of cataracts has also been related to several dietary components, such as vitamin C status (Rawal et al., 1978), and protein deficiency (Bhat, 1983).

To investigate the relationship between nutritional factors and antioxidant defense of the lens of the eye, Jacques et al.. (1988a) conducted a retrospective study of persons with cataracts and matched controls. Serum carotenoid levels were divided into quintiles; in comparison with subjects having moderate carotenoid levels, the group with low levels had four times the risk for developing cataracts. The effect appears to be directly related to carotene level, since the low-serum-carotene group had over 5 1/2 times the risk of developing cataracts as the group with high serum carotenoids. In assessing the results of this study, it must be noted that blood samples were taken after the diagnosis of cataract, and that the relationship between blood and lens concentrations has not been well established (Jacques et al., 1988b). Although the lens contains very little β-carotene, one might propose that the mechanism of β-carotene's protection against cataract formation is through its reduction in the overall oxidative level in the body, and indirectly in the lens. Again, serum β-carotene may represent a marker for the intake of other beneficial components of fruits and vegetables.

IV. SAFETY

β-carotene is absorbed from the intestine with less efficiency as the dietary intake of β-carotene increases. The conversion of β-carotene to vitamin A also declines with increasing β-carotene intake (Goodwin, 1984). The consequence is an increase in circulating β-carotene levels with no significant increase in circulating levels of vitamin A. Therefore, a high intake of β-carotene does not lead to abnormally elevated levels of vitamin A.

Animal studies show that β-carotene is not mutagenic, carcinogenic, or embryotoxic (Heywood et al., 1985). Serum levels of β-carotene in excess of 0.4 mg/dl (Micozzi et al., 1988) are associated with yellow skin coloring. This is a reversible, benign condition, even in infants (Congdon et al., 1981). Treatment with β-carotene supplements at very high levels (up to 150 mg/day) did not cause any toxicity or ophthalmological changes in erythropoietic protoporphyria patients (DeVries–DeMol et al., 1974). There have been reports of amenorrhea associated with high intakes of carotenes (from foods only), but a causal relationship has not been shown (Kemmann et al., 1983). The safety of β-carotene supplementation at doses of 15–50 mg/day has been demonstrated in numerous clinical trials (Bendich, 1988b).

V. SUMMARY

Free radical and singlet oxygen–initiated attack of vital cell components, mutations, and immunosuppression have been implicated in the progression of various chronic diseases. The ability of β-carotene to suppress or counteract these potentially harmful processes may have health implications unrelated to its provitamin A function.

Specific structural features enable β-carotene to be one of the most effective naturally occurring quenchers of singlet oxygen, a highly reactive chemical species. β-carotene is also capable of behaving as an antioxidant and scavenges free radicals generated by reactions other than those involving singlet oxygen. The antimutagenic properties of β-carotene have been demonstrated in studies of individuals who chew excessive amounts of snuff and betel nuts.

The pioneering studies of Mathews-Roth, and the many studies that have followed, have demonstrated the effectiveness of β-carotene therapy for individuals with some light-sensitive skin disorders. In particular, the improvement of patients with erythropoietic porphyria after receiving β-carotene therapy is quite dramatic.

β-carotene enhances immune system function in experimental models. It has been shown to increase T– and B–lymphocyte activity and to enhance tumor rejection in animals.

An overwhelming number of studies have demonstrated that β-carotene may reduce the risk of cancer, particularly lung cancer. In epidemiological studies, a strong association between low β-carotene status and greater cancer risk has been reported for cancer of the bladder, breast, gastrointestinal tract, cervix, esophagus, lung, oropharynx/head and neck, and stomach, primarily of the squamous cell type. The most significant pattern is that seen between high β-carotene intake/status and lower risk of lung cancer.

β-Carotene appears to play a protective role in cataract formation. The mechanism of this effect is unknown.

β-Carotene is a safe substance. At high levels of intake, β-carotene can cause harmless and reversible yellow skin coloration. No toxic dose has been reported.

REFERENCES

Abels, J. C., Gorham, A. T., Pack, G. T., and Rhoads, G. P. (1941). Metabolic studies in patients with cancer of the gastrointestinal tract. I. Plasma vitamin A levels in patients with malignant neoplastic diseases, particularly of the gastrointestinal tract. *J. Clin. Invest.* 20:749–764.

Alexander, M., Newmark, H., and Miller, R. G. (1985). Oral β-carotene can increase the number of OKT4+ cells in human blood. *Immunol Lett.* 9:221–224.

Atukorala, S., Basu, T. K., Dickerson, J. W., Donaldson, D., and Sakula, A. (1979). Vitamin A, zinc and lung cancer. *Br. J. Cancer 40*: 927–931.

Baart de la Faille, H. and Remme, J. J. (1979). Congenital porphyria (Gunther). *Br. J. Dermatol. 101*:224–226.

Basu, T. K., Raven, R. W., Dickerson, J. W., and Williams, D. C. (1974). Vitamin A nutrition and its relationship with plasma cholesterol level in the patients with cancer. *Intl. J. Vit. Nutr. Res 44*: 14–18.

Basu, T. K., Temple, N. J., and Ng, J. (1987). Effect of dietary β-carotene on hepatic drug–metabolizing enzymes in mice. *J. Clin. Biochem. Nutr. 3*:95–102.

Bendich, A. (1988a). A role for carotenoids in immune function. *Clin. Nutr. 7*: 113–117.

Bendich, A. (1988b). The safety of β-carotene. *Nutr. Cancer 11*: 207–214.

Bendich, A. and Shapiro, S. (1986). Effect of β-carotene and canthaxanthin on the immune responses of the rat. *J. Nutr. 116*:2254–2262.

Bhat, K. S. (1983). Distribution of HMW proteins and crystallins in cataractous lenses from undernourished and well–nourished subjects. *Exp. Eye Res. 37*:267–271.

Bond, G. G., Thompson, F. E., and Cook, R. R. (1987). Dietary vitamin A and lung cancer: results of a case–control study among chemical workers. *Nutr. Cancer 9*:109–121.

Brock, K., Berry, G., Mock, P. A., MacLennan, R., Truswell, A. S., and Brinton, L. A. (1988). Nutrients in diet and plasma and risk of in situ cervical cancer. *J. Natl. Cancer Inst. 80*:580–585.

Brown, L. M., Blot, W. J., Schuman, S. H., Smith, V. M. , Ershow, A. G., Marks, R. D., Fraumeni, J. F., Jr. (1988). Environmental factors and high risk of esophageal cancer among men in coastal South Carolina. *J. Natl. Cancer Inst. 80*:1620-1625.

Buiatti, E., Palli, D., Decarli, A., Amadori, D., Avellini, C., Bianchi, S., Biserni, R., Ciprani,F., Cocco, P., Giacosa, A., Marubini, E., Puntoni, R., Vindigni, C., Fraumeni, J., and Blot, W. (1989). A case-control study of gastric cancer and diet in Italy. *Int. J. Cancer 44*:611-616.

Burton, G. W. & Ingold, K. U. (1984). Beta carotene: An unusual type of lipid antioxidant. *Science 224*:569–573.

Byers, T. E., Graham, S., Haughey, B. P., Marshall, J. R., Swanson, M. K. (1987). Diet and lung cancer risk: Findings from the Western New York diet study. *Am. J. Epidemiol 125*:351–363.

Chow, C. K., Thacker, R. R., Changchit, C., Bridges, R. B., Rehm, S. R., Humble, J.,Turbeck, J. (1986). Lower levels of vitamin C and carotenes in plasma of cigarette smokers. *J. Am. Coll. Nutr. 5*:305–312.

Clifford, P. (1972). Carcinogenesis in the nose and throat: nasopharyngeal carcinoma in Kenya. *Proc. R. Soc. Med. 65*:24–28.

Colditz, G. A., Branch, L. G., Lipnick, R. J., Willett, W. C., Rosner, B., Posner, B. M., Hennekens, C. H. (1985). Increased green and yellow

vegetable intake and lowered cancer deaths in an elderly population. *Am. J. Clin. Nutr. 41*:32–36.

Congdon, P. J., Kelleher, J., Edwards, P., and Littlewood,
J. M. (1981). Benign carotenaemia in children. *Arch. Dis. Child
56*:292–294.

Connett, J. E., Kuller, L. H., Kjelsberg, M. O., Polk, B. F., Collins, G.,
Rider, A., and Hulley, S. B. (1989). Relationship between carotenoids
and cancer: the Multiple Risk Factor Intervention Trial (MRFIT)
Study. *Cancer 64*:126–134.

Davis, C., Brittain, E, Hunninghake, D., Graves, K., Buzzard, M. and
Tyroler, H. (1983). Relation between cigarette smoking and serum
vitamin A and carotene in candidates for the Lipid Research Clinics
Coronary Prevention Trial. *Am J. Epidemiol. 118*:445.

Decarli, A., Liati, P., Negri, E., Franceschi, S., La Vecchia, C. (1987). Vitamin A and other dietary factors in the etiology of esophageal cancer. *Nutr. Cancer 10*:29–37.

DeVries–DeMol, E. C., Went, L. N., and Volker–Dieben, H. J. (1974).
Farnsworth–Munsell 100–hue results in a series of patients with
long–standing therapeutic carotenaemia. *Mod. Probl. Ophthalmol.
13*:349–352.

Fontham, E. T. H., Pickle, L. W., Haenszel, W., Correa, P., Lin, Y., and
Falk, R. T. (1988). Dietary vitamins A and C and lung cancer risk in
Louisiana. *Cancer 62*:2267–2273.

Foote, C. S., Denny, R. W., Weaver, L., Chang, Y., Peters,
J. (1970). Quenching of singlet oxygen. *Ann. NY Acad. Sci.
171*:139–148.

Fusaro, R. M. and Johnson, J. A. (1980). Hereditary polymorphic light
eruption in American Indians. *J. Am. Med. Assoc. 244*:1456–1459.

Garewal, H. Allen, V., Killen, D., Elletson, H., Reeves, D., King, D., and
Meyskens, F. (1989). Beta carotene (BC) is an effective, non-toxic
agent for the treatment of premalignant lesions of the oral cavity. *Proc.
Am. Soc. Clin. Oncol. 8*:167.

Gey, K. F., Brubacher, G. B., and Stahelin, H. B. (1987). Plasma levels of
antioxidant vitamins in relation to ischemic heart disease and cancer. *Am J. Clin. Nutr. 45*:1368–1377.

Goodwin, T. W. (1984). Mammals. In *The Biochemistry of the Carotenoids. Vol. II: Animals* Chapman and Hall, New York pp. 173–195.

Graham, S. (1983). Results of case–control studies of diet and cancer in
Buffalo, New York. *Cancer Res. 43*:2409–2413.

Haenszel, W., Correa, P., Lopez, A., Cuello, C., Zarama, G., Zavala, D., and
Fontham, E. (1985). Serum micronutrient levels in relation to gastric
pathology. *Intl. J. Cancer 36*:43–48.

Harris, R. W. C., Forman, D., Doll, R., Vessey, M. P., Wald, N. J. (1986). Cancer of the cervix uteri and vitamin A. *Br. J. Cancer* 53:653–659.

Heywood, R., Palmer, A. K., Gregson, R. L., and Hummler, H. (1985). The toxicity of β-carotene. *Toxicol.* 36:91–100.

Hinds, M. W., Kolonel, L. N., Hankin, J. H., and Lee, J. (1984). Dietary vitamin A, carotene, vitamin C and risk of lung cancer in Hawaii. *Am. J. Epidemiol.* 119:227–237.

Hirayama, T. (1979). Diet and cancer. *Nutr. Cancer* 1:67–81.

Holst, P. A., Kromhout, D., and Brand, R. 1988. For debate: pet birds as an independent risk factor for lung cancer. *Br. Med. J.* 297:1319-1321.

Hu, J., Zhang, S., Jia, E., Wang, Q., Liu, S. , Liu, Y., Wu, Y. and Cheng, Y. (1988). Diet and cancer of the stomach: a case-control study in China. *Intl. J. Cancer* 41:331–335.

Humble, C. G., Samet, J. M., and Skipper, B. E. (1987). Use of quantified and frequency indices of vitamin A intake in a case–control study of lung cancer. *Intl. J. Epidemiol.* 16:341–346.

Jacques, P. F., Chylack, L. T., Jr., McGandy, R. B., and Hartz, S. C. (1988b). Antioxidant status in persons with and without senile cataract. *Arch. Opthalmol.* 106:337–340.

Jacques, P. F., Hartz, S. C., Chylack, L. T., Jr., McGandy, R. B., and Sadowski, J. A. (1988a). Nutritional status in persons with and without senile cataract: blood vitamin and mineral levels. *Am. J. Clin. Nutr.* 48:152–158.

Katsouyanni, K., Willett, W., Trichopoulos, D., Boyle, P., Trichopoulos, A., Vasilaros, S., Papadiamantis, J., and MacMahon, B. (1988). Risk of breast cancer among Greek women in relation to nutrient intake. *Cancer* 61:181–185.

Kemmann, E., Pasquale, S. A., and Skaf, R. (1983). Amenorrhea associated with carotenemia. *J. Am. Med. Assoc.* 249:926–929.

Kobza, A., Ramsay, C. A. and Magnus, I. A. (1973). Oral beta carotene therapy in actinic reticuloid and solar urticaria. *Br. J. Dermatol.* 88:157–166.

Kono, S., Ikeda, M., Tokudome, S., and Kuratsune, M. (1988). A case–control study of gastric cancer and diet in northern Kyushu, Japan. *Jpn. J. Cancer Res.* 79:1067–1074.

Koo, L. C. (1988). Dietary habits and lung cancer risk among Chinese females in Hong Kong who never smoked. *Nutr. Cancer* 11:155–172.

Kromhout, D. (1987). Essential micronutrients in relation to carcinogenesis. *Am. J. Clin. Nutr.* 45:1361-1367.

Kune, G. A. and Kune, S. (1987). The nutritional causes of colorectal cancer. *Nutr. Cancer* 9:1–4.

Kune, G. A. Kune, S., Watson, L. F., Pierce, R., Field, B., Vitetta, L., Merenstein, D., Hayes, A., and Irving, L. (1989). Serum levels of β-carotene, vitamin A, and zinc in male lung cancer cases and controls. *Nutr. Cancer 12*:169–176.

Kvale, G., Bjelke, E., and Gart, J. J. (1983). Dietary habits and lung cancer risk. *Intl. J. Cancer 31*:397–405.

LaVecchia, C., Decarli, A., Franceschi, S., Gentile, A., Negri, E., and Parazzini, F. (1987a). Dietary factors and the risk of breast cancer. *Nutr. Cancer 10*:205–214.

LaVecchia, C., Decarli, A., Fasoli, M., and Gentile, A. (1986). Nutrition and diet in the etiology of endometrial cancer. *Cancer 57*:1248–1253.

LaVecchia, C., Franceschi, S., Decarli, A., Gentile, A., Fasoli, M., Pampallona, S., and Tognoni, G. (1984). Dietary vitamin A and the risk of invasive cervical cancer. *Intl. J. Cancer 34*:319–322.

LaVecchia, C., Negri, E., Decarli, A., D'Avanzo, B., and Francheschi, S. (1987b). A case–control study of diet and gastric cancer in northern Italy. *Intl. J. Cancer 40*:484–489.

LaVecchia, C., Negri, E., Decarli, A., D'Avanzo, B., Gallotti, L., Gentile, A., and Franceschi, S. (1988b). A case–control study of diet and colorectal cancer in northern Italy. *Intl. J. Cancer 41*:492–498.

LaVecchia, C., Negri, E., Decarli, A., D'Avanzo, B., Liberati, C., and Franceschi, S. (1989). Dietary factors in the risk of bladder cancer. *Nutr. Cancer 12*:93–101.

LaVecchia, C., Negri, E., Decarli, A.,Fasoli, M., Parazzini, F.,Franceschi, S., Gentile, A. and Negri, E. (1988a). Dietary vitamin A and the risk of intraepithelial and invasive cervical neoplasia. *Gynecol. Oncol. 30*:187-195.

LeMarchand, L., Yoshizawa, C. N., Kolonel, L. N., Hankin, J. H., and Goodman, M. T. (1989). Vegetable consumption and lung cancer risk: a population–based case–control study in Hawaii. *J. Natl. Cancer Inst. 81*:1158–1164.

MacLennan, R., Da Costa, J., Day, N. E., Law, C. H., Ng, Y. K., Shanmugaratnam, K. (1977). Risk factors for lung cancer in Singapore Chinese, a population with high female incidence rates. *Intl. J. Cancer 20*:854–860.

Marshall, J. R., Graham, S., Byers, T., Swanson, M., and Brasure, J. (1983). Diet and smoking in the epidemiology of cancer of the cervix. *J. Natl. Cancer Inst. 70*:847–851.

Marubini, E., Decarli, A., Costa, A., Mazzoleni, C., Andreoli, C., Barbieri, A., Capitelli, E., Carlucci, M., Cavallo, F., Monferroni, N., Pastorino, U., and Salvini, S. (1988). The relationship of dietary intake and serum levels of retinol and β-carotene with breast cancer: results of a case–control study. *Cancer 61*:173–180.

Mathews–Roth, M. M. (1986). β-carotene therapy for erythropoietic protoporphyria and other photosensitivity diseases. *Biochimie 68*:875–884.

Mathews–Roth, M. M., Pathak, M. A., Fitzpatrick, T. B., Harber, L. H., and Kass, E. H. . (1977). β-carotene therapy for erythropoietic protoporphyria and other photosensitivity diseases. *Arch. Dermatol. 113*:1229–1232.

Mathews–Roth, M. M., Pathak, M. A., Fitzpatrick, T. B., Harber, L. C. and Kass, E. H. (1974). β-carotene as an oral photoprotective agent in erythropoietic protoporphyria. *J. Am. Med. Assoc. 228*:1004–1008.

Mathews–Roth, M. M., Pathak, M. A., Fitzpatrick, T. B., Harber, L. C., and Kass, E. H. (1970). β-carotene as a photoprotective agent in erythropoietic protoporphyria. *N. Engl. J. Med 282*:1231–1234.

Menkes, M. S., Comstock, G. W., Vuilleumier, J. P., Helsing, K. J., Rider, A. A. and Brookmeyer, R. (1986). Serum β-carotene, vitamins A and E, selenium, and the risk of lung cancer. *N. Engl. J. Med. 315*:1250–1254.

Mettlin, C. (1989). Milk drinking, other beverage habits, and lung cancer risk. *Int. J. Cancer 43*:608–612.

Mettlin, C., Graham, S., and Swanson, M. (1979). Vitamin A and lung cancer. *J. Natl. Cancer Inst. 62*:1435–1438.

Micozzi, M. S., Brown, E. D., Taylor, P. R., and Wolfe, E. (1988). Carotenodermia in men with elevated carotenoid intake from foods and β-carotene supplements. *Am. J. Clin. Nutr. 48*: 1061–1064.

Modan, B., Cuckle, H., and Lubin, F. (1981). A note on the role of dietary retinol and carotene in human gastro–intestinal cancer. *Intl. J. Cancer 28*:421–424.

Nierenberg, D. W., Stukel, T. A., Baron, J. A., Dain, B. J., Greenberg, E. R., and The Skin Cancer Prevention Study Group. (1989). Determinants of plasma levels of beta-carotene and retinol. *Am. J. Epidemiol. 130*:511–521.

Nomura, A. M., Stemmermann, G., Heilbrun, L. K., Salkeld, R. M., and Vuilleumier, J. P. (1985). Serum vitamin levels and the risk of cancer of specific sites in Hawaiian males of Japanese ancestry. *Cancer Res. 45*:2369–2372.

Norell, S. E., Ahlbom, A., Erwald, R., Jacobson, G., Lindberg–Navier, I., Olin, R., Tornberg, B., and Wiechel, K. L. (1986). Diet and pancreatic cancer: a case–control study. *Am. J. Epidemiol. 124*:894–902.

Orr, J. W., Wilson, K., Bodiford, C., Cornwell, A., Soong, S. J., Honea, K. L., Hatch, K. D., and Shingleton, H. M. (1985). Corpus and cervix cancer: A nutritional comparison. *Am. J. Obstet. Gynecol. 153*: 775–779.

Paganini–Hill, A., Chao, A., Ross, R. K., and Henderson, B. E. (1987). Vitamin A, β-carotene, and the risk of cancer: a prospective study. *J. Natl. Cancer Inst. 79*:443–448.

Palan, P. R., Romney, S. L., Mikhail, M., Basu, J., and Vermund, S. H. (1988). Decreased plasma β-carotene levels in women with uterine cervical dysplasias and cancer. *J. Natl. Cancer Inst. 80*: 454–455.

Parrish, J. A., Le Vine, M. J., Morrison, W. L., Gonzalez, E., and Fitzpatrick, T. B. (1979). Comparison of PUVA and β-carotene in the treatment of polymorphous light eruption. *Br. J. Dermatol. 100*: 187–193.

Pastorino, U., Pisani, P., Berrino, F., Andreoli, C., Barbieri, A., Costa, A., Mazzoleni, C., Gramegna, G., and Marubini, E. (1987). Vitamin A and female lung cancer: a case–control study on plasma and diet. *Nutr. Cancer 10*:171–179.

Pisani, P., Berrino, F., Macaluso, M., Pastorino, U., Crosignani, P. and Baldassaroni, A. (1986). Carrots, green vegetables and lung cancer: A case control study. *Intl. J. Epidemiol. 15*:463–468.

Rawal, W. M., Patel, U. S., and Desai, R. J. (1978). Biochemical studies on cataractous human lenses. *Indian J. Med. Res. 67*:161–164.

Rohan, T. E., McMichael, A. J., and Baghurst, P. A. (1988). A population–based case–control study of diet and breast cancer in Australia. *Am. J. Epidemiol. 128*:478–489.

Russell–Briefel, R., Bates, M. W., and Kuller, L. H. (1985). The relationship of plasma carotenoids to health and biochemical factors in middle–aged men. *Am. J. Epidemiol. 122*:741–749.

Samet, J. M., Skipper, B. J., Humble, C. G., and Pathak, D. R. (1985). Lung cancer risk and vitamin A consumption in New Mexico. *Am. Rev. Respir. Dis. 131*:198–202.

Santamaria, L., Bianchi, A., Mobilio, G., Santagati, G., Ravetto, C., Bernardo, G., and Vetere, C. (1988). Cancer chemoprevention by carotenoids: experimental evidence and human interventions after radical surgery. In *Nutrition, Growth and Cancer,* G. P. Tryfiates and K. N. Prasad (Eds.). Alan R. Liss, New York, pp. 177–200.

Schrott, E. L. (1985). Carotenoids in plant photoprotection. *Pure and Appl. Chem. 57*:729–734.

Schwartz, J. and Shklar, G. (1987). Regression of experimental hamster cancer by β-carotene and algae extracts. *J. Oral Maxillofac. Surg. 45*:510–515.

Schwartz, J. and Shklar, G. (1988). Regression of experimental oral carcinomas by local injection of β-carotene and canthaxanthin. *Nutr. Cancer 11*:35–40.

Schwartz, J. Suda, D., and Light, G. (1986). β-carotene is associated with the regression of hamster buccal pouch carcinoma and the induction of tumor necrosis factor in macrophages. *Biochem. Biophys. Res. Comm. 136*:1130–1135.

Seifter, E., Rettura, G., Padawer, J., Stratford, F., Goodwin, P., and Levenson, S. M. (1983). Regression of C3HBA mouse tumor due to x–ray therapy combined with supplemental β-carotene or vitamin A. *J. Natl. Cancer Inst. 71*:409–417.

Seifter, E., Rettura, G., Padawer, J., Stratford, F., Weinzweig, J., Demetriou, A. A., and Levenson, S. M. (1984). Morbidity and mortality reduction by supplemental vitamin A or β-carotene in CBA mice given total–body gamma–irradiation. *J. Natl. Cancer Inst. 73*: 1167–1177.

Shekelle, R., Liu, S., Raynor, W., Lepper, M., Maliza, C., Rossof, A., Paul, O., Shryock, A., Stamler, J. (1981). Dietary vitamin A and risk of cancer in the Western Electric study. *Lancet 2*:1185–1189.

Sistrom, W. R., Griffith, M. Stanier, R. Y. (1956). The biology of a photosynthetic bacterium which lacks colored carotenoids. *J. Cell. Comp. Physiol. 48*:473–515.

Slattery, M. L., Sorenson, A. W., Mahoney, A. W., French, T. K., Kritchevsky, D., and Street, J. C. (1988). Diet and colon cancer: assesment of risk by fiber type and food source. *Natl. Cancer Inst. 80*:1474-1480.

Sneddon, I. B. (1974). Congenital porphyria. *Proc. R. Soc. Med. 67*: 593–594.

Stich, H. F., Stich, W., Rosin, M., Vallejera, M. (1984). Use of the micronucleus test to monitor the effect of vitamin A, β-carotene and canthaxanthin on the buccal mucosa of betel nut/tobacco chewers. *Intl. J. Cancer 34:745–750.*

Stich, H. F., Hornby, A. P., Dunn, B. P. (1985). A pilot β-carotene intervention trial with Inuits using smokeless tobacco. *Intl. J. Cancer 36*:321–327.

Stich, H. F., Hornby, A. P., Dunn, B. (1986). β-carotene levels in exfoliated mucosa cells of population groups at low and elevated risk for oral cancer. *Intl. J. Cancer 376*:389–393.

Stich, H. F., Rosin, M. P., Hornby, A. P., Mathew, B., Sankaranarayanan, R. , and Nair, M. K. (1988). Remission of oral leukoplakias and micronuclei in tobacco/betel quid chewers treated with β-carotene plus vitamin A. *Intl. J. Cancer 42:*195-199.

Stryker, W. S., Kaplan, L. A., Stein, E. A., Stampfer, M. J., Sober, A., and Willett, W. C. (1988). The relation of diet, cigarette smoking, and alcohol consumption to plasma β-carotene and alpha–tocopherol levels. *Am J. Epidemiol. 127*:283–296.

Stryker, S., Stein, E. A., Kaplan, L., Stampfer, M., Sober, A. and Willett, W. C. (1987). Effects of diet, alcohol and cigarette use on the blood levels of β-carotene. *J. Am. Coll. Nutr. 6*:73.

Thomsen, K., Schmidt, H., Fischer, A. (1979). β-carotene in erythropoietic protoporphyria: 5 years experience. *Dermatologica 159*:82–86.

Tomita, Y., Hlmeno, K., Nomoto, K., Endo, H., and Hirohata, T. (1987). Augmentation of tumor immunity against syngeneic tumors in mice by β-carotene. *J. Natl. Cancer Inst. 78*:679–681.

Tomkin, G. H., Scott, L., Ogbuah, C., and Oshaughnessy, M. (1986). Carcinoma of the colon–association with low dietary vitamin A in females: preliminary communication. *J. Roy. Soc. Med. 79*:462–464.

Tuyns, A. J., Riboli, E., Doornbos, G., and Pequignot, G. (1987). Diet and esophageal cancer in Calvados (France). *Nutr. Cancer 9*:81–92.

Varma, S. D., Chand, D., Sharma, Y. R.,, Kuck, J. F., and Richards, R. D. (1984). Oxidative stress on lens and cataract formation: role of light and oxygen. *Current Eye. Res. 3*:35–57.

Verreault, R., Chu, J., Mandelson, M., and Shy, K. (1989). A case–control study of diet and invasive cervical cancer. *Int. J. Cancer 43*:1050–1054.

Wahi, P. N., Bodhke, R. R., Arora, S., and Sriustaua, M. C. (1962). Serum vitamin A studies in leukoplakia and carcinoma of the oral cavity. *Indian J. Pathol. Bacteriol. 5*:10–16.

Wald, N. J., Boreham, J., Hayward, J. L., and Bulbrook, R. D. (1984). Plasma retinol, β-carotene, and vitamin E levels in relation to the future risk of breast cancer. *Br J. Cancer 49*:321–324.

Wald, N. J., Thompson, S. G., Densem, J. W., Boreham, J., and Bailey, A. (1988). Serum β-carotene and subsequent risk of cancer: results from the BUPA study. *Br. J. Cancer 57*:428–433.

West, D. W., Slattery, M. L., Robison, L. M., Schuman, K. L., Ford, M. H., Mahoney, A. W., Lyon, J. L., and Sorenson, A. W. (1989). Dietary intake and colon cancer: sex– and anatomic site-specific associations. *Am. J. Epidemiol. 130*:883-894.

Willett, W., Polk,·B. F., Underwood, B., Stampfer, M. J., Pressel, S., Rosner, B., Taylor, J., Schneider, K., Hames, C. G. (1984). Relation of serum vitamins A and E and carotenoids to the risk of cancer. *N. Eng. J. Med. 310*:430–434.

Winn, D. M., Ziegler, R. G., Pickle, L. W., Gridley, G., Blot, W. J., and Hoover, R. N. (1984). Diet in the etiology of oral and pharyngeal cancer among women from the southern United States. *Cancer Res.* 44:1216–1222.

Witter, F. R., Blake, D. A., Baumgardner, R., Mellits, E. D., and Niebyl, J. R. (1982). Folate, carotene and smoking. *Am. J. Obstet. Gynecol. 144*:857.

Wu, A. H., Henderson, B. E., Pike, M. C. and Yu, M. C. (1985). Smoking and other risk factors for lung cancer in women. *J. Natl. Cancer Inst.* 74:747–751.

Wu, A. H., Paganini–Hill, A., Ross, R. K., and Henderson, B. E. (1987). Alcohol, physical activity and other risk factors for colorectal cancer: a prospective study. *Br. J. Cancer 55*:687–694.

Wylie–Rosett, J. A., Romney, S. L., Slagle, S., Wassertheil–Smoller, S., Miller, G. L., Palan, P., Lucido, D. J., and Duttagupta, C. (1984). Influence of vitamin A on cervical dysplasia and carcinoma in situ. *Nutr. Cancer 6*:49–57.

Young, T. B. and Wolf, D. A. (1988). Case–control study of proximal and distal colon cancer and diet in Wisconsin. *Intl. J. Cancer 42*:167–175.

You, W. C., Blot, W. J., Chang, Y. S., Ershow, A. G., Yang, Z. T., An, Q., Henderson, B., Xu, G. W., Fraumeni, J. F., and Wang, T. G. (1988). Diet and high risk of stomach cancer in Shandong, China. *Cancer Res. 48*:3518–3523.

Ziegler, R. G., Mason, T. J., Stemhagen, A., Hoover, R., Schoenberg, J. B., Gridley, G., Virgo, P., and Fraumeni, J. (1986). Carotenoid intake, vegetables, and the risk of lung cancer among white men in New Jersey. *Am. J. Epidemiol. 123*:1080–1091.

Ziegler, R. G., Morris, L. E., Blot, W. J., Pottern, L. M., Hoover, R., and Fraumeni, J. F. (1981). Esophageal cancer among black men in Washington, D. C. : Role of nutrition. *J. Natl. Cancer Inst.* 67:1199–1205.

4

Vitamin D

S. K. Gaby and V. N. Singh

I. INTRODUCTION

Vitamin D is a prohormone and in a classical sense is not an essential nutrient. However, a specific deficiency disease has been associated with inadequate vitamin D intake, and it has been traditionally classified as a vitamin. The endogenous provitamin, 7–dehydrocholesterol, and ergocalciferol (vitamin D_2), the form used in food fortification, are converted to cholecalciferol (vitamin D_3) by radiation. This conversion takes place in skin exposed to sunlight or to an artificial source of ultraviolet light.

A. Metabolism and Function

Dietary vitamin D is absorbed in the same manner as other lipids, and with about a 50% efficiency (Miller and Norman, 1984). After being taken up by the liver, both the vitamin D_2 and vitamin D_3 forms circulate in the blood attached to a vitamin D-binding protein. The major storage sites are adipose tissue and muscle (Mawer et al.,1972).

The most widely recognized vitamin D function is its role in the maintenance of calcium and phosphorus homeostasis. Vitamin D enhances calcium and phosphorus absorption and promotes bone formation. Vitamin D_3 is converted to $25(OH)D_3$ in the liver. The conversion to $1,25(OH)_2D_3$ takes place in the kidney. Blood and dietary calcium levels, as well as

59

parathyroid hormone (PTH) regulate renal 1–hydroxylase, the metabolic control point for producing $1,25(OH)_2D_3$, the most active form of vitamin D. The function of another active metabolite of vitamin D, $24,25(OH)_2D_3$, remains unclear, but it appears to be important in ossification.

The roles of vitamin D in mammalian reproduction (Halloran, 1989; Kwiecinski et al., 1989), immune function (Provvedini et al., 1983; Gray and Cohen, 1985; Manolagas et al., 1989), and gene regulation (Shapiro et al., 1989) are the focus of current research. Vitamin D is thought to function in a manner similar to other steroid hormones, that is, by entering the nucleus of target cells and activating RNA synthesis.

Beneficial therapeutic effects of both oral intake and topical application of vitamin D and vitamin D analogs in psoriasis have been reported (Kato et al., 1986; Morimoto et al., 1986; Takamoto et al., 1986; Kragballe et al., 1988; Smith et al., 1988). This finding is consistent with the discovery of vitamin D receptors on skin cells (Colston et al., 1981; Holick et al., 1987) and the reported influence of the metabolites on cellular differentiation (Abe et al., 1981; Hosomi et al. 1983).

B. Deficiency and Sources

Rickets, the disease caused by poor vitamin D status in children, is characterized by bowed legs, spinal curvature, joint enlargement, and stress–induced deformities of the ribs and pelvis. In adults, vitamin D deficiency results in osteomalacia, which can cause bone pain and muscle weakness. Both conditions are the result of bone loss.

Fish liver oils and salt water fish are the only rich dietary sources of vitamin D. Small amounts of the nutrient are present in other animal foods. Plant foods are extremely poor sources of vitamin D. In the United States, the major sources of dietary vitamin D are fortified foods such as milk. The U.S. Recommended Daily Allowance (RDA) for vitamin D is 400 IU (10 μg cholecalciferol) for all healthy people.

C. Special Vitamin D Needs of the Elderly

Elderly people in the United States may be at risk of having poor vitamin D status. A number of factors contribute to this risk: decreased exposure to sunlight, especially in northern areas, decreased caloric intake, intake of vitamin D fortified dairy products, decreased absorption of nutrients, and, for some individuals, decreased 1–hydroxylase activity in the kidney. In addition, in vitro studies suggest that when exposed to sun, the skin of elderly people produces less than half the vitamin D produced by the skin of young people (MacLaughlin and Holick, 1985).

Although the efficiency of absorption of vitamin D was found to vary widely among individuals, healthy elderly subjects appear to absorb vitamin D as efficiently as younger subjects (Guillemant et al., 1982). Also, age per se does not appear to reduce renal hydroxylation of 25(OH)D3 (Aksnes et al., 1989). These findings suggest that poor intake combined with low exposure to sunlight and restricted synthesis in the skin may be principally responsible for low vitamin D status in older individuals. Many elderly people in developed countries are at risk of developing osteomalacia (Barzel, 1983). Moderate vitamin D supplementation is considered reasonable prophylaxis (Grueter et al., 1987; Webb and Holick, 1988), and may consequently decrease the risk of bone fractures.

In addition to osteomalacia, "marginal" hypovitaminosis D may contribute to bone brittleness in the elderly. Older subjects in the Netherlands who had hip fractures were found to have poorer vitamin D status than controls of the same age, although vitamin D intake was low for all subjects (Lips et al., 1987).

In a group of healthy elderly French people, all were found to have vitamin D intakes of less than 5 μg/day (200 IU), with reduced serum calcium and 25(OH)D3 levels and elevated PTH (Chapuy et al., 1987). Supplementation with calcium and ergocalciferol (20 μg/day) increased calcium and 25(OH)D3 levels, and reduced PTH. Thus, in apparently healthy people, supplementation ameliorated signs of secondary hyperparathyroidism, which has been associated with an increased risk of bone fractures.

D. Risk of Inadequate Vitamin D Status

In addition to the elderly, infants may also require supplemental vitamin D, since human milk does not contain vitamin D at a level considered to provide for optimal growth (Committee on Dietary Allowances, 1980) and because liver and kidney function may be inadequate, especially in premature and low birth weight infants.

Diseases affecting fat absorption, the liver, kidneys, or thyroid may cause secondary vitamin D deficiency. Individuals consuming a vegetarian diet without supplemental vitamin D, particularly individuals with dark skin pigmentation and those with little sun exposure, may also be at risk for frank or marginal hypovitaminosis D.

II. HEALTH BENEFITS

A. Reducing Osteoporosis Risk

Intestinal absorption of calcium is dependent on 1,25(OH)2D3, so that an inadequate supply of vitamin D, low sunlight exposure, or renal insufficiency can result in reduced absorption of calcium. Low serum calcium stimulates PTH secretion, which mobilizes calcium from bones. Vitamin D deficiency is associated with hyperparathyroidism and bone loss. As discussed, this may be a particular problem for the elderly.

The association between vitamin D and bone health has been explored in epidemiological studies, which have yielded ambiguous results. A large number of intervention trials, primarily with postmenopausal women as subjects, have been conducted in the area of vitamin D and prevention of osteoporotic degeneration. In some studies, vitamin D analogs have been shown to increase dietary calcium absorption (Gallagher et al., 1979, 1982; Lawoyin et al., 1980). Other studies have found only a transient increase in absorption (Reeve et al., 1982) or no change (Lindholm and Eriksson, 1982). Improving absorption of calcium may be necessary, but perhaps insufficient, to slow or reverse osteoporosis. In addition, postmenopausal subjects who already have signs of osteoporosis may not be the best population for intervention trials. Premenopausal women have a greater ability to absorb calcium, and it may be very difficult to affect bone mass in postmenopausal women. Prevention of osteoporosis may therefore require early intervention, establishing a healthy bone mass before menopause (Spencer and Kramer, 1986).

Various methods have been used to quantitate the effects of calcium and/or vitamin D treatment on bone loss. In one study, bone biopsy (the most direct measurement), showed that supplementation with vitamin D and calcium increased bone formation and mineralization (Lund et al., 1975). Forearm x–ray showed an apparent reduction in the rate of bone loss in one trial (Nordin et al., 1985), but no effect of treatment in another (Jensen et al., 1982). Using somewhat more subjective measurements, subjects with painful spinal crush fractures were found to have significantly less pain than controls following supplementation with vitamin D, calcium and fluoride (Grove and Halver, 1981).

An analysis of fractures in nursing home residents suggested that risk of bone fracture increased with low circulating levels of $1,25(OH)_2D_3$, but risk was not reduced by normal levels of $25(OH)D_3$ (Rudman et al., 1989). The increased fracture risk was thus attributed to impaired renal hydroxylation, not to an inadequate vitamin D status.

Although vitamin D analogs have been shown to be useful in many of these trials, the findings are inconsistent and do not currently justify widespread use of these agents in the treatment of osteoporosis (Parfitt, 1988). The complex etiology of osteoporosis suggests that a single agent would not be a very effective prophylaxis. Vitamin D is one of a number of factors necessary to optimize bone health.

B. Cardiovascular Health

High blood pressure is considered an important risk factor for cardiovascular disease (CVD). Epidemiological and intervention trials have shown an inverse relationship between blood pressure (BP) and calcium status and/or intake (Belizan et al., 1983; McCarron et al., 1982, 1984; Ljunghall et al., 1987). There are several mechanisms by which calcium has been postulated to lower blood pressure: a reduction in parathyroid hormone production, reduction in intracellular calcium concentration (an effect associated with the antihypertensive effects of calcium entry blockers, β blockers and diuretics), and an alteration in smooth muscle contraction (Ljunghall et al., 1987). Calcium metabolism is regulated by several factors, including parathyroid hormone, calcitonin (thyrocalcitonin), and vitamin D.

In early studies, it had been suggested that individuals with CVD were producing or ingesting higher amounts of vitamin D than other individuals (Knox, 1973; Linden, 1974). An analysis of serum from patients who had had a myocardial infarction (MI) showed that their vitamin D status was normal, and that vitamin D was not correlated with certain other postulated CVD risk factors: triglycerides, cholesterol, calcium, or magnesium levels (Lund et al., 1978). If vitamin D status is causally related to CVD, either positively or negatively, it may be through calcium and/or magnesium (Seelig, 1975) metabolism. However, such a relationship was not seen in the study of subjects who have had an MI (Lund et al., 1978) and has not been clearly demonstrated elsewhere.

An age–adjusted inverse relationship between dietary vitamin D and systolic BP was reported in women aged 20–35 years (Sowers et al., 1985). In older women (55–80 years) in the same study, this inverse relationship was maintained only if the subjects' consumption of both calcium and vitamin D was below the U.S. RDA (Sowers et al., 1985).

In one study, serum levels of $1,25(OH)_2D_3$ were found to be positively associated with diastolic and systolic BP in a cohort of normotensive and hypertensive older women, when adjusted for age, weight, and diuretic use (Sowers et al., 1988). The trend was not significant in premenopausal women. The authors theorized that an increase in the level of the vitamin may be a response to low plasma ionized calcium; this may represent a homeostatic mechanism for increasing calcium and reducing hypertension. Both blood pressure and $1,25(OH)_2D_3$ would therefore remain high in refractory cases. High circulating levels of $1,25(OH)_2D_3$ have also been reported in hypertensives with low renin activity (Resnick et al., 1986), implying a possible relationship between the hormones regulating calcium and sodium metabolism, and between those hormones and blood pressure.

Calcium intake has been negatively associated with the incidence of hypertension (McCarron et al., 1984). In an intervention trial, neither calcium supplementation nor combined calcium and 1,25(OH)$_2$D$_3$ supplementation had a significant effect on arterial pressure in essential hypertension (Zoccali et al., 1988). However, the vitamin was administered to only eight subjects, and for only two weeks, so that the finding of no effect may be considered inconclusive. Vitamin D analogs have been found to reduce hypertension in intervention trials (Lind et al., 1987, 1988), notably in low-renin hypertension (Lind et al., 1989).

Several studies have reported an association between vitamin D and/or calcium status and hypertension; in addition, vitamin D analogs have been shown to be potentially valuable in the treatment of some forms of hypertension. It remains to be seen whether a beneficial effect on BP can be derived from increased dietary or supplemental vitamin D.

C. Reducing Cancer Risk

Vitamin D has been shown to inhibit carcinogenesis and the growth of cancer cells in animal models (Eisman et al., 1987; Pence and Buddingh, 1988; Colston et al., 1989; Kawaura et al., 1989). Preliminary work suggests that there may be a role for vitamin D in reducing the risk of some types of human cancer.

In the Western Electric study, a 19–year prospective dietary intake survey, risk of mortality from colorectal cancer was inversely correlated with both vitamin D and calcium consumption (Garland et al., 1985). In a second prospective study, blood samples were taken from a population of 25,620 individuals (Garland et al., 1989). Levels of 25(OH)D$_3$ were measured in samples from 34 individuals who later developed colon cancer and from 67 controls. A serum concentration of 20 ng/ml or more was associated with one-third the risk of developing colon cancer that was associated with lower concentrations of 25(OH)D$_3$. In another study, longer healthy survival times were reported for subjects who had mammary tumors with 1,25(OH)$_2$D$_3$ receptors than for subjects whose tumors were receptor–negative (Colston et al., 1989). This suggests the possibility of in vivo inhibition of cancerous cells by vitamin D, as is seen in vitro (Rossi et al., 1988).

While these findings are promising, a body of clinical evidence for an anticarcinogenic effect of vitamin D is currently lacking.

III. SAFETY

Vitamin D is an extremely potent agent. Hypervitaminosis D, which is associated primarily with high levels of the (unbound) metabolite 25(OH)D$_3$, is a potentially serious condition and can cause permanent kidney damage, growth retardation, hypercalcemia, calcification of soft tissues, and death. Mild symptoms of vitamin D intoxication are nausea, weakness, constipation, and irritability. Adverse reactions to vitamin D have been reported for intakes as low as 25,000 IU/day, although daily intakes below 50,000 IU are not thought to cause toxicity in most adults (Miller and Hayes, 1982). These levels are 62–125 times higher than the U.S. RDA of 400 IU. However, some infants and individuals with hypercalcemia are more sensitive to vitamin D. Vitamin D intake for these individuals should not exceed 2000 IU/day (Miller and Hayes, 1982). Vitamin D production from sunlight exposure is self–limiting, so that overexposure to sun will not cause hypervitaminosis D in healthy people.

Large doses of vitamin D and its synthetic analogs are clearly teratogenic in animals (Nebel and Ornoy, 1972; McClain et al., 1980; Ornoy et al., 1980; Zusman and Ornoy, 1981). Based on the assumption that the same may be true for humans, intakes of vitamin D greatly in excess of the U.S. RDA are not recommended for pregnant women.

IV. SUMMARY

Vitamin D is a prohormone traditionally classified as a vitamin. It is known to be critical for bone maintenance and the absorption and metabolism of calcium and phosphorus.

Elderly people, infants, vegetarians, individuals with limited ultraviolet light absorption (due to skin pigmentation and/or sun exposure), and people with certain medical conditions may be at risk of poor vitamin D status.

Epidemiological evidence indicates that adequate vitamin D status can reduce the risk of osteoporosis.

Vitamin D, presumably via calcium metabolism, appears to play some role in regulating blood pressure. Good vitamin D status and treatment with vitamin D analogs have been associated with improvement of some forms of hypertension.

There is suggestive, but very preliminary, evidence that vitamin D may have an anticarcinogenic function, particularly in colon cancer.

Vitamin D can be very toxic at extremely high intakes. No adverse effects in healthy adults have been reported for consumption up to about 62 times the U.S. RDA. Vitamin D is teratogenic in animal models; intakes by women of childbearing potential should be limited to U.S. RDA levels.

REFERENCES

Abe, E., Miyaura, C., Sakagami, H., Takeda, M., Konno, K., Yamazaki, T., Yoshiki, S., and Suda, T. (1981). Differentiation of mouse myeloid leukemia cells induced by 1-alpha, 25-dihydroxyvitamin D₃. *Proc. Natl. Acad. Sci. USA* 78:4990–4994.

Aksnes, L., Rodland, O., Odegaard, O. R., Bakke, K. J., and Aarskog, D. (1989). Serum levels of vitamin D metabolites in the elderly. *Acta Endocrinol. (Copenh.)* 121:27–33.

Barzel, U. S. (1983). Vitamin D deficiency: a risk factor for osteomalacia in the aged. *J. Am. Geriatr. Soc.* 31:598–601.

Belizan, J. M., Villar, J., Pineda, O., Gonzalez, A. E., Sainz, E., Garrera, G., and Sibrian, R. (1983). Reduction of blood pressure with calcium supplementation in young adults. *J. Am. Med. Assoc.* 249:1161–1165.

Chapuy, M. C., Chapuy, P., and Meunier, P. J. (1987). Calcium and vitamin D supplements: effects on calcium metabolism in elderly people. *Am. J. Clin. Nutr.* 46:324–328.

Colston, K., Colston, M. J., and Feldman, D. (1981).1,25-Dihydroxyvitamin D₃ and malignant melonoma: the presence of receptors and inhibition of cell growth in culture. *Endocrinology 108*:1083–1086.

Colston, K. W., Berger, U., and Coombes, R. C. (1989). Possible role for vitamin D in controlling breast cancer cell proliferation. *Lancet 1*:188–191.

Committee on Dietary Allowances, Food and Nutrition Board (1980). *Recommended Dietary Allowances,* 9th rev. ed. National Academy of Sciences, Washington DC.

Eisman, J. A., Barkla, D. H., and Tutton, P. J. M. (1987). Suppression of in vivo growth of human cancer solid tumor xenografts by 1,25-dihydroxyvitamin D3. *Cancer Res.* 47:21–25.

Gallagher, J. C., Riggs, B. L., Eisman, J., Hamstra, A., Arnaud, S. B., and DeLuca, H. F. (1979). Intestinal calcium absorption and serum vitamin D metabolites in normal subjects and osteoporotic patients: effect of age and dietary calcium. *J. Clin. Invest.* 64:729–736.

Gallagher, J. C., Jerpabak, C. M., Jee, W. S. S., Johnson, K. A., DeLuca, H. F., and Riggs, B. L. (1982). 1,25-Dihydroxyvitamin D₃: short- and long-term effects on bone and calcium metabolism in patients with postmenopausal osteoporosis. *Proc. Natl. Acad. Sci. USA 79*: 3325–3329.

Garland, C., Barrett-Connor, E., Rossof, A. H., Shekelle, R. B., Criqui, M. H., and Paul, O. (1985). Dietary vitamin D and calcium and risk of colorectal cancer: a 19-year prospective study in men. *Lancet 1*:307–309.

Garland, C. F., Garland, F. C., Shaw, E. K., Comstock, G. W., Helsing, K. J., and Gorham, E. D. (1989). Serum 25-hydroxyvitamin D and colon cancer: eight-year prospective study. *Lancet* 2:1176–1178.

Gray, T. K. and Cohen, M. S. (1985). Vitamin D, phagocyte differentiation and immune function. *Surv. Immunol. Res.* 4:200– 212.

Grove, O. and Halver, B. (1981). Relief of osteoporotic backache with fluoride, calcium and calciferol. *Acta Med. Scand.* 209:469– 471.

Grueter, J., Marmet, J., Keagy, E., Rehm, W., Kretz, A., and Kunovits, G. (1987). Vitamin D supplementation in the elderly. *Lancet* 1:306–307.

Guillemant, S., Prier, A., Guillemant, J., Massin, J. P., and Camus, J. P. (1982). Absorption et métabolisme de la vitamine D3 marquée chez le sujet agé. *Rev. Rhumatisme* 49:93–98.

Halloran, B. P. (1989). Is 1,25-dihydroxyvitamin D required for reproduction? *Proc. Soc. Exp. Biol. Med.* 191:227–232.

Holick, M. F., Smith, E., and Pincus, S. (1987). Skin as the site of vitamin D synthesis and target tissue for 1,25-dihydroxyvitamin D3. *Arch. Dermatol.* 123:1677–1683a.

Hosomi, J., Hosoi, J., Abe, E., Suda, T., and Kuroki, T. (1983). Regulation of terminal differentiation of cultured mouse epidermal cells by 1-alpha, 25-dihydroxyvitamin D3. *Endocrinology* 113:1950–1957.

Jensen, G. F., Christiansen, C., and Transbol, I. (1982). Treatment of post menopausal osteoporosis. A controlled therapeutic trial comparing oestrogen/gestagen, 1,25-dihydroxy-vitamin D3 and calcium. *Clin. Endocrinol.* 16:515–524.

Kato, T., Rokugo, M., Terui, T., and Tagami, H. (1986). Successful treatment of psoriasis with topical application of active vitamin D3 analogue, 1-alpha, 24-dihydroxycholecalciferol. *Br. J. Dermatol.* 115:431–433.

Kawaura, A., Tanida, N., Sawada, K., Oda, M., and Shimoyama, T. (1989). Supplemental administration of 1-alpha-hydroxyvitamin D3 inhibits promotion by intrarectal instillation of lithocholic acid in N-methyl-N-nitrosourea-induced colonic tumorigenesis in rats. *Carcinogenesis* 10:647–649.

Knox, E. G. (1973). Ischaemic heart disease mortality and dietary intake of calcium. *Lancet* 1:1465–1467.

Kragballe, K., Beck, H. I., and Sogaard, H. (1988). Improvement of psoriasis by a topical vitamin D3 analogue (MC 903) in a double-blind study. *Br. J. Dermatol.* 119:223–230.

Kwiecinski, G. G., Petrie, G. I., and DeLuca, H. F. (1989). Vitamin D is necessary for reproductive functions of the male rat. *J. Nutr.* 119:741–744.

Lawoyin, S., Zerwekh, J. E., Glass, K., and Pak, C. Y. C. (1980). Ability of 25-hydroxyvitamin D3 therapy to augment serum 1,25- and 24, 25-dihydroxyvitamin D in postmenopausal osteoporosis. *J. Clin. Endocrinol. Metab. 50*:593–596.

Lind, L., Wengle, B., and Ljunghall, S. (1987). Blood pressure is lowered by vitamin D (alphacalcidol) during long-term treatment of patients with intermittent hypercalcaemia. *Acta Med. Scand. 222*:423–427.

Lind, L., Lithell, H., Skarfors, E., Wide, L., and Ljunghall, S. (1988). Reduction of blood pressure by treatment with alphacalcidol: a double-blind, placebo-controlled study in subjects with impaired glucose tolerance. *Acta Med. Scand. 223*:211–217.

Lind, L., Wengle, B., and Ljunghall, S. (1989). Reduction of blood pressure during long-term treatment with active vitamin D (alphacalcidol) is dependent on plasma renin activity and calcium status: a double-blind, placebo-controlled study. *Am. J. Hypertens. 2*:20–25.

Linden, V. (1974). Vitamin D and myocardial infarction. *Br. Med. J. 3*:647–650.

Lindholm, T. S. and Eriksson, S. (1982). Bone mineral and calcium metabolism before, during and after treatment of osteoporosis with 1-alpha-hydroxyvitamin D3 and calcium. *Scand. J. Rheumatol. 11*:55–57.

Lips, P., van Ginkel, F. C., Jongen, M. J. M., Rubertus, F., van der Vijgh, W. J. F., and Netelenbos, J. C. (1987). Determinants of vitamin D status in patients with hip fracture and in elderly control subjects. *Am. J. Clin. Nutr. 46*:1005–1010.

Ljunghall, S., Hvarfner, A., and Lind, L. (1987). Clinical studies of calcium metabolism in essential hypertension. *Eur. Heart J. 8*:37–44.

Lund, B., Kjaer, I., Friis, T., Hjorth, L., Reimann, I., Andersen, R. B., and Sorensen, O. H. (1975). Treatment of osteoporosis of ageing with 1-alpha-hydroxycholecalciferol. *Lancet 2*:1168–1171.

Lund, B., Badskjaer, J., Lund, B., and Soerensen, O. H. (1978). Vitamin D and ischaemic heart disease. *Horm. Metab. Res. 10*:553–556.

MacLaughlin, J. and Holick, M. F. (1985). Aging decreases the capacity of human skin to produce vitamin D3. *J. Clin. Invest. 76*:1536–1538.

Manolagas, S. C., Hustmyer, F. G., and Yu, X. P. (1989). 1,25-Dihydroxyvitamin D3 and the immune system. *Proc. Soc. Exp. Biol. Med. 191*:238–245.

Mawer, E. B., Backhouse, J., Holman, C. A., Lumb, G. A., and Stanbury, S. W. (1972). The distribution and storage of vitamin D and its metabolites in human tissues. *Clin. Sci. 43*:413–431.

McCarron, D. A. (1982). Low serum concentrations of ionized calcium in patients with hypertension. *N. Engl. J. Med. 307*:226–228.

McCarron, D. A., Morris, C. D., Henry, H. J., and Stanton, J. L. (1984). Blood pressure and nutrient intake in the United States. *Science* 224:1392–1398.

McClain, R. M., Langhoff, L., and Hoar, R. M. (1980). Reproduction studies with 1-alpha-25-dihydroxyvitamin D3 (calcitriol) in rats and rabbits. *Toxicol. Appl. Pharmacol.* 52:89–98.

Miller, B. E. and Norman, A. W. (1984). Vitamin D. In *Handbook of Vitamins: Nutritional, Biochemical, and Clinical Aspects*, L. J. Machlin (Ed.). Marcel Dekker, New York, pp. 45–97.

Miller, D. R. and Hayes, K. C. (1982). Vitamin excess and toxicity. In *Nutritional Toxicology*, vol. 1, J. N. Hathcock, (Ed.). Academic Press, New York, pp. 81–133.

Morimoto, S., Yoshikawa, K., Kozuka, T., Kitano, Y., Imanaka, S., Fukuo, K., Koh, E., and Kumahara, Y. (1986). An open study of vitamin D3 treatment in psoriasis vulgaris. *Br. J. Dermatol.* 115:421–429.

Nebel, L. and Ornoy, A. (1972). Interdependence of fetal anomalies and placental impairment following maternal hypervitaminosis D and hypercortisonism. In *Drugs and Fetal Development*, M. A. Klingberg, A. Abramovici, and J. Chemke, (Eds.). Plenum Press, New York, pp. 251–255.

Nordin, B. E. C., Baker, M. R., Horsman, A., and Peacock, M. (1985). A prospective trial of the effect of vitamin D supplementation on metacarpal bone loss in elderly women. *Am. J. Clin. Nutr.* 42:470–474.

Ornoy, A., Hirsch, B. E., Zusman, I., and Atkin, I. (1980). The transplacental effects of vitamin D metabolites and corticosteroids on the long bones of rat and mice fetuses. Teratol Limbs, 4th Symp. Prenatal Dev., pp. 339–354.

Parfitt, A. M. (1988). Use of calciferol and its metabolites and analogues in osteoporosis. *Drugs* 36:513–520.

Pence, B. C. and Buddingh, F. (1988). Inhibition of dietary fat promoted colon carcinogenesis in rats by supplemental calcium or vitamin D. *Carcinogenesis* 9:187–190.

Provvedini, D. M., Tsoukas, C. D., Deftos, L. J., and Manolagas, S. C. (1983). 1,25-dihydroxyvitamin D3 receptors in human leukocytes. *Science* 221:1181–1183.

Reeve, J., Tellez, M., Green, J. R., Hesp, R., Elsasser, U., Wootton, R., Hulme, P., Williams, D., Kanis, J. A., Russell, R. G. G., Mawer, E. B., and Meunier, P. J. (1982). Long-term treatment of osteoporosis with 24, 25 dihydroxycholecalciferol. *Acta Endocrinol.* 101:636–640.

Resnick, L. M., Muller, F. B., and Laragh, J. H. (1986). Calcium regulating hormones in essential hypertension: relation to plasma renin activity and sodium metabolism. *Ann. Intern. Med.* 105:649–654.

Rossi, J. F., Durie, B. G. M., Duperray, C., Braich, T., Marion, S. L., Pike, J. W., Haussler, M. R., Janbon, C., and Bataille, R. (1988). Phenotypic and functional analysis of 1,25-dihydroxyvitamin D3 receptor mediated modulation of the human myeloma cell line RPMI 8226. *Cancer Res.* *48*:1213–1216.

Rudman, D., Rudman, I. W., Mattson, D. E., Nagraj, H. S., Caindec, N., and Jackson, D. L. (1989). Fractures in the men of a veterans administration nursing home: relation to 1,25-dihydroxyvitamin D. *J. Am. Coll. Nutr.* *8*:324–334.

Seelig, M. S. (1975). Ischaemic heart disease, vitamins D and A, and magnesium. *Br. Med. J.* *3*:647–648.

Shapiro, L. H., Venta, P. J., Yu, Y. S. L., and Tashian, R. E. (1989). Carbonic anhydrase II is induced in HL-60 cells by 1,25-dihydroxyvitamin D3: a model for osteoclast gene regulation. *FEBS Lett.* *249*:307–310.

Smith, E. L., Pincus, S. H., Donovan, L., and Holick, M. F. (1988). A novel approach for the evaluation and treatment of psoriasis. *J. Am. Acad. Dermatol.* *19*:516–528.

Sowers, M. R., Wallace, R. B., and Lemke, J. H. (1985). The association of intakes of vitamin D and calcium with blood pressure among women. *Am. J. Clin. Nutr.* *42*:135–142.

Sowers, M. R., Wallace, R. B., Hollis, B. W., and Lemke, J. H. (1988). Relationship between 1,25-dihydroxyvitamin D and blood pressure in a geographically defined population. *Am. J. Clin. Nutr.* *48*:1053–1056.

Spencer, H. and Kramer, L. (1986). NIH consensus conference: osteoporosis: factors contributing to osteoporosis. *J. Nutr.* *116*:316–319.

Takamoto, S., Onishi, T., Morimoto, S., Imanaka, S., Yukawa, S., Kozuka, T., Kitano, Y., Seino, Y., and Kumahara, Y. (1986). Effect of 1-alpha-hydroxycholecalciferol on psoriasis vulgaris: a pilot study. *Calcif. Tissue Int.* *39*:360–364.

Webb, A. R. and Holick, M. F. (1988). The role of sunlight in the cutaneous production of vitamin D3. *Annu. Rev. Nutr.* *8*:375–399.

Zoccali C., Mallamaci, F., Delfino, D., Ciccarelli, M., Parlongo, S., Iellamo, D., Moscato, D., and Maggiore, Q. (1988). Double-blind randomized, crossover trial of calcium supplementation in essential hypertension. *J. Hypertens.* *6*:451–455.

Zusman, I. and Ornoy, A. (1981). Transplacental effects of vitamin D3 metabolites on bone formation in rat fetuses. *Isr. J. Med. Sci.* *17*:1191–1192.

5

Vitamin E

S. K Gaby and L. J. Machlin

I. INTRODUCTION

Vitamin E refers to a group of fat-soluble compounds (tocopherols and tocotrienols) with similar biological roles. α-Tocopherol is the most biologically active form. Vitamin E is an essential nutrient for all mammalian species that have been studied. It is required to prevent deficiency symptoms in humans, such as reduced red blood cell lifespan, neuromuscular deficits, and abnormal platelet activity.

The vitamin E molecule is ideally suited to the environment of cellular membranes. Membranes contain a large amount of fatty acids (lipids), which are susceptible to oxidation, especially polyunsaturated fatty acids (PUFAs). One of the principal functions of vitamin E is thought to be the protection of membranes from oxidative damage.

A. Absorption, Transport and Storage

Approximately 20–40% of dietary vitamin E is absorbed from a normal diet; absorption is enhanced by dietary fat. The efficiency of absorption declines as intake increases. Because bile and pancreatic secretions are required, biliary obstruction will seriously impair vitamin E absorption. Vitamin E esters are hydrolyzed in the duodenal mucosa. The vitamin is pre-

71

sumed to be incorporated into micelles with other lipids and transferred across membranes by as yet uncharacterized diffusion.

Vitamin E circulates bound to lipoproteins and in red blood cells. The vitamin E level in blood is highly correlated with total serum lipids. Principal storage depots for vitamin E are adipose tissue, liver, and muscle. The highest concentrations of the vitamin are in the adrenal and pituitary glands, testes, platelets, and heart, although vitamin E has been shown to accumulate in all tissues of animals when consumed in high quantities.

B. Requirements and Dietary Sources

Vitamin E deficiency disease is rarely seen except in starvation and conditions where fat absorption is limited, such as premature birth, biliary atresia, short bowel syndrome and cystic fibrosis. The U.S. Recommended Daily Allowance for vitamin E is 30 IU (10 α-tocopherol equivalents).

Vitamin E is present in small quantities in a large number of foods. The richest sources are wheat germ oil, vegetable oils, egg yolk, nuts, green plants, milk fat, and liver.

II. ANTIOXIDANT FUNCTION

Vitamin E is the primary fat-soluble antioxidant (see Introduction) and the principal means of breaking free radical chain reactions in most tissues (Ingold et al., 1987).

Vitamin E can protect critical cellular structures against damage both from free radicals (such as peroxy radical, hydroxyl radical, and superoxide) and from oxidation products, (such as malondialdehyde and hydroxynonenal), which also have deleterious effects. Malondialdehyde causes undesirable bonding of lipids and of proteins (Tappel, 1973). These bonds, or cross-links, prevent the molecules from functioning normally. Cross-linking can affect membrane proteins (Tappel, 1974) and chromosomes (Cutler, 1976).

Pentane is produced from the oxidative breakdown of omega-6 fatty acids such as linoleic acid, and pentane measurement is therefore useful as a marker of lipid peroxidation (Pincemail et al., 1987). Pentane exhalation was found to be negatively correlated with vitamin E status, and was lowered by a daily supplementation of 1000 IU for ten days (Lemoyne et al., 1987). Another trial, with 400 mg/day vitamin E or placebo, showed that a group of mountaineers receiving the vitamin for 4 weeks did not increase their pentane production while climbing. Controls increased pentane exhalation by more than 100% (Simon-Schnass et al., 1987). These studies suggest that there is a measurable, in vivo, protective antioxidant effect of vitamin E.

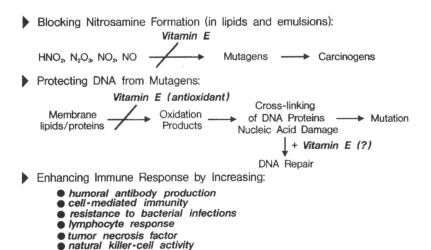

▶ Blocking Nitrosamine Formation (in lipids and emulsions):

▶ Protecting DNA from Mutagens:

▶ Enhancing Immune Response by Increasing:
  - *humoral antibody production*
  - *cell-mediated immunity*
  - *resistance to bacterial infections*
  - *lymphocyte response*
  - *tumor necrosis factor*
  - *natural killer-cell activity*

Figure 1   Possible mechanisms of Vitamin E protection against cancer induction.

III. HEALTH BENEFITS

A. Cancer Risk

Vitamin E, as an important antioxidant, plays a role in immunocompetence, inhibition of mutagen formation, and repair of membranes and DNA. Because of the probable association between these functions and inhibition of carcinogenesis, it has been suggested that vitamin E may be useful in cancer prevention (Newmark and Mergens, 1981; Bright-See and Newmark, 1983; London et al., 1985a). Proposed mechanisms of vitamin E protection against cancer induction are shown in Figure 1.

1.   Animal Models

One way in which vitamin E may inhibit carcinogenesis is through stimulation of the immune system. Vitamin E administration to hamsters resulted in regression of chemically induced tumors (Shklar et al., 1987), possibly due to the concomitant stimulation of tumor necrosis factor-alpha (Shklar and Schwartz, 1988). However, vitamin E showed no immunoenhancement in a study of chemically induced tumors in the rat (Ip and White, 1987).

2.   Nitrosamines and Vitamin E

Vitamin E has been shown to block the formation of nitrosamines (Mergens et al., 1978; Mirvish 1986). Nitrosamines can be mutagenic and carcinogenic. They are formed in the body and in foods and cigarette smoke from nitrates and nitrites reacting with amines, compounds that occur naturally in foods and in the body.

Although no causal relationship has been established between the prevalence of nitrosamines in the gut and cancers of the gastrointestinal tract, studies have been conducted to investigate whether or not supplemental vitamin E can reduce nitrosamines and other fecal mutagens. Dion and others (1982) found that in cases where fecal mutagenicity was present, a 400 mg daily supplement of each of the vitamins C and E for 2 weeks reduced mutagenicity by 75%. A 500 mg supplement of vitamin E reduced nitrosamine levels in urine by about 50% when nitrosation was experimentally induced in one human subject (Ohshima and Bartsch, 1981), but was less effective than vitamin C (a water soluble antioxidant).

3.   Cancer and Vitamin E Levels

Several researchers have measured the blood concentration of vitamin E in individuals with cancer or precancerous conditions (Tables 1 and 2). In an ongoing study of gastric cancer in a group of Colombian men, serum vitamin E levels were found to be lower in subjects with gastric dysplasia (a precancerous condition) than in men with less severe abnormalities or with normal stomach cells (Haenszel et al., 1985). It is not clear whether low vitamin E status predisposes these subjects to gastric dysplasia or whether the differences in vitamin E status are a consequence of the pathology (through either metabolic change or impaired absorption). The blood concentration of vitamin E in ovarian cancer patients was not different from that of controls (Heinonen et al., 1985). On the other hand, serum vitamin E concentration was significantly lower in individuals with advanced lung cancer than in controls; vitamin E levels were also significantly lower in the offspring of the lung cancer patients (Miyamoto et al., 1987). This suggests that the difference in nutritional status may not be entirely explained by metabolic changes associated with the disease state.

4.   Cancer and Vitamin E: Prospective Epidemiological Studies

Eight prospective studies were conducted in which blood samples were collected from very large groups of people and stored (Tables 1 and 2). During subsequent years cancer cases were identified and the blood levels of vitamin E from the stored samples were compared with those of matched controls without cancer. In a group of Finnish men the relative risk for developing cancer was 0.64 for men with vitamin E levels in the upper two quintiles, compared to a relative risk of 1 for those with levels in the three lower

Table 1   Epidemiological Studies of Vitamin E and Cancer

Authors	Year	Findings related to serum vitamin E
Effect of vitamin E found		
Wald et al.	1984	Lowest levels associated with a five-fold increase in breast cancer risk, compared with highest levels
Haenszel et al.	1985	Low levels in subjects with (precancerous) gastric dysplasia
Salonen et al.	1985	Low vitamin E and selenium levels, but not low vitamin E alone, were associated with increased risk of fatal cancer
Menkes et al.	1986	Lowest quintile associated with a 2.5 relative risk of developing lung cancer, compared with subjects having highest serum level
Kok et al.	1987	Lowest quintile level associated with a four-fold increased risk of developing some type of cancer compared with highest quintile.
Miyamoto et al.	1987	Levels significantly lower in lung cancer patients and their offspring
Knekt et al.	1988	Low levels associated with increased risk of developing cancer
No effects found		
Stahelin et al.	1984	Low levels in men who later developed colon cancer, but the difference was not significant[a]
Willett et al.	1984	Levels 8% lower in subjects who later developed cancer, but the difference was not significant[a]
Nomura et al.	1985	No association with later incidence of cancers of the lung, stomach, colon, rectum, or urinary bladder
Heinonen et al.	1985	No difference in level between ovarian tumor cases and controls
Wald et al.	1987	No association between level and later development of cancer
Russell et al.	1988	No association between level and later development of breast cancer

[a]Differences in blood lipid levels may account for most of the difference between groups.

Table 2   Summary of Epidemiological Studies of Serum Vitamin E and Cancer

Reference	Site of cancer	Mean difference in serum Vitamin E (μg/ml) (cases minus controls)	Statistical significance	Relative risk lowest vs. highest
Prospective studies				
Wald et al., 1984	Breast	−1.3	p < 0.025	5
Willett et al., 1984	All	−1.0	N.S.	–
Menkes et al., 1986	Lung	−1.4	p < 0.001	2.5
Salonen et al., 1985	All	−0.1	N.S.	–
Nomura et al., 1985	5 sites	0.0	N.S.	–
Stahelin et al., 1984	All	−0.9	N.S.	–
Wald et al., 1987	All	−0.2	N.S.	
Wald et al., 1987	All above studies	−0.43	p = 0.003	
Kok et al., 1987	Lung	−0.8	N.S.	–
	All	−1.3	p < 0.005	4.4
Knekt et al., 1988	All	−0.3	p < 0.05	1.56
Retrospective studies (serum levels of cases measured after diagnosis)				
Haenszel et al., 1985	Gastric dysplasia	−1.2	p < 0.05	
Heinonen et al., 1985	Ovary	−1.1	N.S.	
Miyamoto et al., 1987	Lung	−3.1	p < 0.001	
Offspring of lung cancer patients		−1.24	p < 0.05	

N.S. = Not significant.

quintiles (Knekt et al., 1988). Kok and others (1987) found that cancer risk was 4.4 times higher in individuals in the lowest compared to the highest quintile of serum vitamin E. Low serum levels of vitamin E were also associated with increased subsequent risk of breast cancer (Wald et al., 1984), although these results may have been an artifact of poor sample handling (Wald et al., 1988). Low vitamin E in combination with low serum selenium was associated with increased risk of cancer death (Salonen et al., 1985).

Dietary intakes of many nutrients and types of food were estimated in a case-control study of esophageal cancer in France (Tuyns et al., 1985). The relative risk of developing esophageal cancer (adjusted for alcohol and tobacco use) associated with the highest level of vitamin E consumption was less than one-third (0.27) of the risk associated with the lowest intake (Table 3).

Some studies have not found statistically significant differences in vitamin E status between individuals who later developed cancer and those who did not (see Table 2); the data show, however, that the serum vitamin E levels tend to be consistently lower in cases than controls.

No statistically significant association was found between serum vitamin E and subsequent risk of developing cancer in studies of individuals in a hypertension control program (Willett et al., 1984), although the serum level of vitamin E was about 8% lower in those who later developed cancer. Similarly, the lower levels of serum vitamin E in men at risk for cardiovascular diseases who later developed cancer of the colon were not significantly different from those of controls (Stahelin et al., 1984). There was no association between serum vitamin E levels and subsequent risk of breast

Table 3   Effect of β–Carotene and Vitamins E and C on Risk of Esophageal Cancer[a]

Nutrient	Relative risks by consumption level		
	Low	Moderate	High
β-Carotene	1.0	0.85	0.47[b]
Vitamin C	1.0	0.67[b]	0.38[b]
Vitamin E	1.0	0.40[b]	0.27[b]

[a] Adjusted for alcohol and tobacco use.
[b] $p < 0.05$.
Source: Adapted from Tuyns et al., 1985.

cancer development in a group of British women, though serum levels tended to be low in both controls and future cases (Russell et al., 1988). No protective effect from vitamin E against any type of cancer was found in a study of Hawaiian males of Japanese ancestry (Nomura et al., 1985).

Wald and others (1987) found no correlation between serum vitamin E levels and later cancer development, except in cases where the cancer was diagnosed within a year of sample collection. This finding supports the suggestion that vitamin E status declines as a result of cancer. However, in most of the other studies blood samples were collected more than a year before diagnosis. Moreover, in the study of Miyamoto the offspring of lung cancer patients had significantly lower serum vitamin E levels than did individuals in families without a history of lung cancer. Therefore, it is likely that there is an association between a low vitamin E status and subsequent risk of developing some forms of cancer.

5. Current Research

Based on the data correlating low vitamin E status with increased cancer risk, intervention trials are underway (Bertram et al. 1987). These studies are investigating the efficacy of vitamin E supplementation in the prevention of certain cancers.

B. Cardiovascular Disease

1. Platelet Function

In response to an injury to a blood vessel, platelets in the blood stream first adhere to the injured sire and then become "sticky" and clump together (aggregate). During this process the platelets generate chemical signals, prostaglandins. This results in a escalation of the clumping process and eventual thrombosis, which plugs the blood vessel. This is a vital function which prevents an organism from bleeding to death. Nonetheless, there are drawbacks to this platelet response: hyperaggregability, where platelets too readily aggregate, can lead to blood clots, and potentially, myocardial infarcts or stroke; and the sequelae of aggregation can start, or at least contribute to, the development of atherosclerotic plaques (calcification and fatty accumulation in the aggregated clumps) (see Introduction).

Vitamin E and Platelets.   Vitamin E has been shown to inhibit the platelet prostaglandin release reaction in vitro (Steiner and Anastasi, 1976; Fong, 1976). There is also evidence of reduced platelet aggregation in blood samples from volunteers taking very high levels of vitamin E supplements (Steiner, 1983) (Table 4,) although this was not found to be the case in a study of short-term, high-dose supplementation (Huijgens et al., 1981).

Table 4 Experimental Data on High Dose Vitamin E and Platelets in Humans

Subjects	Vitamin E	Duration	Findings	Reference
6 healthy men	2000 IU/ day	10 days	No change in bleeding time, aggregation or platelet prostaglandin synthesis	Huijgens et al., 1981
47 healthy men and women	400, 800, and 1200 IU/day	2 weeks each	Significant decrease in platelet adhesive–ness to collagen	Steiner, 1983
46 patients with hyper–lipoprotein–emias	300 or 600 IU/day[a]	2 weeks	Suppressed elevated plasma lipid peroxides; at 600 mg, mild platelet suppressant effect	Szczeklik et al., 1985
30 women on hormonal contra–ceptives	200 IU/ day[a]	2 months	Decreased platelet activity, decrease in contraceptive–induced increase in clotting	Renaud et al., 1987
9 insulin dependent diabetics	1000 IU/ day	35 days	Decreased ADP–induced platelet aggregation, malondialdehyde release, and TXB_2 production	Colette et al., 1988
10 women and 10 men	800 IU/ day or placebo	5 weeks	No significant differences in platelet aggregation, bleeding time, or prosta–cyclin or TXB_2 production	Stampfer et al., 1988
4 male and 3 female adult nonsmokers	400, 800, 1200 or 1600 IU/ day	2 weeks each dose level	Increased platelet adhesion in vitro to fibrinogen and collagen; no dose–related difference in adhesiveness	Jandak et al., 1988

[a] Crossover placebo trial

During the platelet aggregation process there is an increase in oxidation of arachidonic acid with the formation of prostaglandins such as thromboxane. The antiaggregatory effect of vitamin E may be due to its inhibition of this oxidation or may involve an effect on membrane fluidity (Steiner, 1981; Steiner and Mower, 1982). The mechanism(s) of vitamin E action on platelets is still speculative. In in vitro studies, vitamin E has been shown to inhibit critical enzymes in prostaglandin synthesis, cyclooxygenase (Steiner and Mower, 1982) and lipoxygenase (Gwebu et al., 1980).

The concentration of vitamin E in platelets has been found to decline with age (Vatassery et al., 1983). It has been hypothesized that the platelet hyperactivity and increase in arachidonic acid oxidation (compared with young subjects) found in a group of elderly subjects is causally related to their significantly reduced platelet vitamin E levels (Vericel et al., 1988).

Women using oral contraceptives, who were found to have reduced vitamin E levels and increased platelet clotting, were given vitamin E supplements of 200 mg/day for 2 months. Following supplementation, blood samples from the women showed markedly reduced platelet activity (aggregation and clotting) (Renaud et al., 1987). However, healthy volunteers (who were not taking hormones) supplemented with 800 IU of vitamin E for five weeks showed no significant differences from controls in bleeding time, in thromboxane or prostacyclin synthesis, or in in vitro platelet aggregation response (Stampfer et al., 1988).

When 400 IU/day of vitamin E was given to subjects it strongly inhibited in vitro platelet adhesion to collagen (Steiner, 1983, 1987), fibrinogen, and fibronectin (Jandak et al., 1988). This is significant in that adhesion of platelets to collagen (exposed when the lining of blood vessels is injured) is an important step in the formation of thrombi. This effect would complement the action of potent agents, such as aspirin, that inhibit aggregation but have no effect on adhesion.

Platelets and Vitamin E Intake.   Platelet vitamin E content reflects dietary intake (Lehmann et al., 1988). This finding suggests that changes in vitamin E consumption could alter platelet function in vivo.

Vitamin E, Platelets, and Diabetes.   People with insulin-dependent diabetes mellitus (IDDM) may have increased platelet clotting activity (Colwell et al., 1983), although some workers have found clotting to be normal in subjects with IDDM (Petersen and Gormsen 1978). [The increased activity may be diminished by proper insulin administration (Colwell et al., 1983).] An increased aggregatory rate is seen in diabetics with proliferative retinopathy (Watanabe et al., 1984).

The platelets of diabetics produced more thromboxanes in vitro than those of nondiabetics (Karpen et al., 1984, 1985). This increase in platelet aggregating factors correlated negatively with platelet vitamin E concentrations: low vitamin E was associated with high thromboxane synthesis. A double-blind, crossover placebo study of 9 patients with IDDM treated with 1g of vitamin E /day for 35 days showed significant reduction in platelet aggregation and malondialdehyde release with treatment (Colette et al.,1988). It has been suggested that the increase in platelet aggregation and the synthesis of proaggregatory prostaglandins are contributing factors in the microvascular disease associated with IDDM (for a review, see Colwell et al., 1983).

2.   Intermittent Claudication

Intermittent claudication is the result of various vascular disorders (such as atherosclerosis) which result in insufficient blood flow. This lack of blood to exercised muscles can cause cramping, pain, numbness and fatigue.

The treatment of intermittent claudication with vitamin E supplements has been investigated for many years with mixed results (Housley and McFadyen, 1974). The use of vitamin E appears to be safe, and useful in certain cases (Pinsky, 1980).

An early double-blind placebo study of high-dose vitamin E administration for intermittent claudication showed improvement in 67% of only those subjects who had poor circulation in the lower leg (Williams et al., 1971). A study was carried out by Haeger in which 300 mg/day vitamin E supplementation was accompanied by a cessation of smoking and an increase in exercise (Haeger, 1973). After 2 years the treated group had a 34% increase in arterial flow to the lower leg, with no change in controls receiving dicoumarin (an anticoagulant) or vasodilator drugs. Patient success in passing a distance walking test was 54% in vitamin E-treated vs. 23% in control subjects (Haeger, 1974). Similar results were seen in follow-up studies of the use of vitamin E in long-term treatment for intermittent claudication (Haeger,1978,1982).

3.   Ischemic Reperfusion Injuries

Ischemia (a loss of the blood supply to an area) can cause tissue damage. Alleviation of ischemia when blood supply and therefore oxygen is restored (reperfusion) can further damage tissue by causing an increase in free radical production (see McCord, 1988, for a review). There is substantial evidence that free radical scavengers such as vitamin E are protective against reperfusion injury (Burton, 1988).

Studies using perfused rat heart from α-tocopherol prefed animals (Massey et al., 1986, Chiu et al., 1987) show a significant protective effect of vitamin E. In a study of reperfused rabbit heart, infusion of α-tocopherol protected the muscle from some of the damage associated with ischemia and reperfusion (Ferrari et al., 1987).

Bypass Surgery. Cardiopulmonary bypass surgery involves a temporary cessation of blood flow to the heart, followed by reperfusion, and thus the heart may be subject to ischemia-reperfusion injury (McCord, 1985). Thirty patients undergoing the bypass procedure participated in a study of the effects of vitamin E supplementation on reducing free radical damage to membranes (Cavarocchi et al., 1986). Ten of the subjects received in oral supplement of 2000 IU of vitamin E 12 hours before surgery. The supplemented group showed no significant increase in hydrogen peroxide (H_2O_2) (an indicator of oxidative stress) during the procedure and a significant reduction in H_2O_2 in comparison with controls. The supplement also prevented the significant reduction in serum vitamin E level that was seen in the control subjects 24 hours after surgery. Further studies are necessary to determine whether there is an increased requirement for vitamin E during cardiopulmonary bypass surgery.

4. Ischemic Heart Disease Mortality

In summarizing preliminary data from several epidemiological studies, Gey and others concluded that antioxidant vitamin status, particularly that of vitamin E, is a factor in the relative risk of mortality from ischemic heart disease (IHD). After standardizing for blood lipid levels, low vitamin E status correlated with increased risk of IHD (Gey et al., 1987). In countries with relatively high IHD mortality rates (Scotland and Finland), the plasma vitamin E level was found to be about 25% lower ($p<0.01$) than in countries with low to moderate coronary mortality rates (Italy, Switzerland and Northern Ireland) (see Fig. 2).

C. Immunity and Infection

Vitamin E supplementation has been shown to increase resistance to infection in numerous farm and laboratory animals (Corwin and Gordon, 1982; Meeker et al., 1985; see Tengerdy, 1980, and Bendich, 1987, for reviews). Vitamin E may enhance immune function by inhibiting the production of certain immunosuppressive prostaglandins (Likoff et al., 1981; Lawrence et al., 1985) or moderating granulocyte activation (Lafuze et al., 1984). The protective effect of the vitamin is associated with a reduction in the hydrogen peroxide generated by phagocytic cells of the immune system.

1. Studies in Humans

One retrospective epidemiological study of 100 healthy elderly people found a statistically significant association between high vitamin E status (plasma vitamin E level greater than 1.35 mg/dl) and low incidence of in-

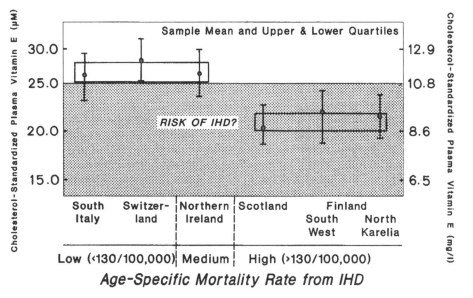

Figure 2   Correlation of plasma vitamin E with ischemic heart disease mortality. Plasma samples from apparently healthy males aged 40–49, (Gey et al.,1987).

fections over a 3-year period (Chavance et al., 1984) (Fig. 3). For most individuals an intake of 40–60 IU/day would be required to maintain a blood level over 1.35 mg/dl (Fig.4). An intervention trial using 200 and 400 mg daily vitamin E supplements for 3 months in 103 adults showed no effect on serum antibody response to a viral vaccine or incidence of infection (Harman and Miller, 1986); however, antibody titers are not indicative of the body's ability to fight viral infections. Also, there were no initial measurements of subjects' vitamin E intake or blood levels (which may have been high), so the change in vitamin E status cannot be determined.

In the only well-controlled double-blind study examining the effects of vitamin E on immune responses, healthy subjects 60 years of age and older had significant improvement in several clinical indicators of immune function. The supplemented group was given 800 IU of vitamin E daily for 1 month and had increased blood levels of α-tocopherol, improved delayed hypersensitivity skin test response, increase interleukin-2 response to mitogens, as well as decreased plasma lipid peroxides (Meydani et al., 1989).

Vobecky et al., (1986b) measured the serum values of several vitamins and minerals as well as immunoglobulin levels (used as an index of immune response) in healthy preschool children. Subjects with serum vitamin E concentrations above the 90th percentile had higher IgG, IgA, and IgM levels, although the difference was not statistically significant (Vobecky et al., 1986b). These investigators also looked at blastogenic indices, an in vitro measure of cell-mediated immunity. The index of response to pokeweed mitogen and tetanus toxoid was significantly higher in children above the 90th percentile in vitamin E status (Vobecky et al., 1986a). The mean blastogenic indices were also higher in this group in response to concanavalin and phytohemagglutinin mitogens, but the difference from the children with a lower vitamin E status was not statistically significant.

An uncontrolled human study showed significant decreases in in vitro bactericidal activity of leukocytes and mitogen induced lymphocyte transformation in eight subjects supplemented with 300 mg vitamin E per day for 3 weeks (Prasad, 1980). Leukocytes employ oxidation to destroy bacteria, and this capacity may be reduced by the antioxidant action of vitamin E. However, there was no change in immunological response associated with vitamin E supplementation as measured by an in vivo test of delayed hypersensitivity (Prasad, 1980). Delayed hypersensitivity is a measure of

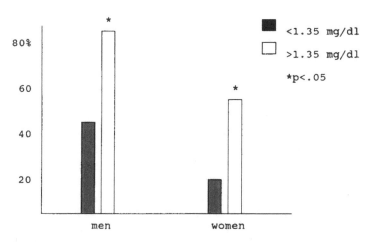

Figure 3   Percent of elderly with no more than two infections over a 3-year period: Relationship to vitamin E status (Chavance et al., 1984.)

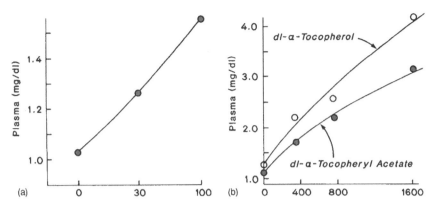

Figure 4   Effect of vitamin E supplements on α–tocopherol concentration in blood (a) Supplemental vitamin E per day (IU) (Lehmann et al., 1988). (b) Supplemental vitamin E per day (IU) (Baker et al., 1980).

the immune response which is more relevant to infection resistance than the in vitro parameters.

Despite a few conflicting reports, the majority of studies in animals and in humans support the suggestion that higher levels of vitamin E are associated with enhanced immune response.

D.   Cataracts

Numerous studies have suggested that cataract development may be related to oxidative stress, particularly when coupled with reduced antioxidant protection in the aging eye. Vitamin E has been shown to reduce significantly the progression of the disorder and damage to the eye in animal models of cataract (Bhuyan et al., 1982; Varma et al., 1984). Antioxidants may also have a protective role against cataract formation in humans (Jacques et al.,1988b; Taylor,1989; see Chapter 3).

A recent human study investigated the relationship between plasma nutrient levels and the incidence of development of several types of cataract (Jacques et al., 1988a). The investigators found a lower risk of posterior subcapsular cataract associated with high plasma vitamin E levels, although the evidence of an effect was not strong (Table 5). However, the combination of high vitamin E status with high blood levels of beta-caro-

Table 5   Relative Risk for Cataract by Level of Antioxidant Vitamins in Blood

Nutrient	Cataract[a]	Lowest quintile	Highest quintile
Carotenoids	NUC	1.0	0.18 p < 0.10
	COR	1.0	0.14 p < 0.05
	PS	1.0	0.18
Vitamin C	NUC	1.0	0.29
	COR	1.0	0.27
	PS	1.0	0.09 p < 0.10
Vitamin E	NUC	1.0	0.83
	COR	1.0	0.84
	PS	1.0	0.33

[a] NUC = nuclear; COR = cortical; PS = posterior subcapsular.
Source : Adapted from Jacques et al., 1988a.

tene and/or vitamin C was associated with a significant decrease in risk of developing cataracts (Jacques et al., 1988b) (Table 6).

Daily supplementation with 400 IU of vitamin E was correlated with a 0.40 relative risk of having a cataract, compared with a relative risk of 1 among those who did not report taking a supplement, in a study of 175 people with cataracts and 175 controls (Robertson et al., 1989) (Table 7).

Evidence from animal and human studies supports a role for vitamin E in the prevention of cataracts. Further investigation is necessary to con-

Table 6   Effect of Antioxidant Vitamins E and C and β–Carotene on Relative Risk of Cataracts

	Vitamin Status[a]		
	Low[b]	Middle	High[b]
Relative risk	1.0	0.6	0.2 (p < 0.05)

[a] 77 cases and 35 controls aged 40–70 years.
[b] Low = subject is in the lowest quintile in at least one vitamin and not in the highest quintile for either of the other vitamins. High = subject is in the highest quintile for at least two vitamins and is not in the lowest quintile for the other vitamin.
Source: Data from Jacques et al., 1988b.

Table 7   Effect of Vitamins E and C Supplements on Risk of Cataract in People over 55 Years Old

Supplement	Relative risk	
None	1.00	
Vitamin E (400 IU)	0.40	p = 0.003
Vitamin C (300–600 mg)	0.25	p = 0.04
Vitamin E and C	0.32	p = 0.05

Source: Data from Robertson et al., 1989.

firm the efficacy of vitamin E supplementation in reducing the risk of cataract formation in humans.

E. Exercise

Vitamin E supplementation of athletes has produced equivocal effects on performance (Helgheim et al., 1979). The current consensus, based on well-controlled research, is that vitamin E supplementation does not improve athletic performance (Farrell, 1980). However, vitamin E may play an important role in preventing exercise–induced muscle injury.

In the rat, adaptation to exercise training includes a significant increase in the levels of antioxidant enzymes within cells and a decreased tissue concentration of vitamin E (Quintanilha, 1984). Additional animal studies have suggested that exercise increases free radical reactions in tissues and is associated with an increased metabolism of vitamin E (Packer 1984; Gohil et al., 1987). In humans vitamin E is mobilized during heavy exercise, possibly as a result of the breakdown of fat stores (Pincemail et al., 1988).

There also appears to be an increased antioxidant demand in exercising humans. The changes in lipid peroxidation during exercise have been estimated through the measurement of exhaled pentane (Tappel and Dillard 1981) (see section II of this chapter.). Healthy subjects who received 1200 IU/day of α-tocopherol for 2 weeks had significantly lower pentane production while resting and exercising than nonsupplemented controls (Dillard et al., 1978). While pentane production more than doubled in a placebo control group of high-altitude mountain climbers, a group supplemented with 400 mg α-tocopherol per day showed no significant change in pentane exhalation (Simon-Schnass et al., 1987). Thus, under some circumstances vitamin E may protect muscle from the damaging effects of exercise-induced free radical injury.

F. Fibrocystic Breast Disease

Fibrocystic breast disease is a benign, though often painful condition resulting from excessive growth of connective tissue. The course and development of the disease are related to estrogen and progesterone levels, and to a subsequent increased risk of breast cancer (see Vorherr, 1986, for a review).

Sundaram and others (1981) conducted a study with 26 patients and 5 controls who received a 2×300 mg/day α-tocopherol supplement for 2 months (following 1 month of placebo supplementation). Objective and subjective remission was achieved in 85% of the patients after treatment. The same laboratory did not find evidence of a beneficial effect of the vitamin in a larger, more controlled study (London et al., 1985b). Another group of investigators found a similar lack of efficacy in treatment of fibrocystic breast disease with vitamin E (Ernster et al., 1985).

G. Neurological Disorders

Neurological abnormalities are associated with vitamin E deficiency (Muller et al., 1983; Harding, 1987). Neuropathic and myopathic symptoms have been documented and shown to respond to vitamin E repletion in humans (Howard et al., 1982; Sokol, 1989). The mechanism of action of vitamin E is assumed to be through antioxidant protection of membranes and/or membrane stabilization. It has been suggested that the large surface area of certain neurons is particularly susceptible to oxidative damage (Muller, 1986).

Current research in the etiology of neurological disorders such as Alzheimer's disease and Parkinson's disease suggests that environmental factors play an important role in initiating the disease years before symptoms appear (Calne et al., 1986). It has been theorized that oxidative damage caused by these environmental factors may be involved in the development of parkinsonism, and that antioxidants such as vitamin E may be effective in early treatment of the disease (Cadet ,1986; Grimes et al., 1987). Although animal studies of chemically induced parkinsonism show no improvement or prevention with high-dose vitamin E administration (Russ et al., 1987), a preliminary human trial was encouraging (Fahn, 1989). Factor and Weiner found that patients with Parkinson's disease who were self-supplementing with vitamin E had significantly less severe disease than matched controls (1989).

Tardive dyskinesia is a disorder caused by long-term use of certain neuroleptic drugs. The uncontrolled movements associated with the disorder may be the result of oxidation damage to nerve endings (Cadet et al., 1986). A cross-over placebo study of 15 patients with tardive dyskinesia was conducted with 1200 IU of α-tocopherol for 2-week periods (Lohr et al., 1987). The supplemented group exhibited a 43% reduction in scores of an abnormal involuntary movement test. Control scores were not changed significantly. Further research would be desirable to establish whether there is a role for vitamin E supplementation in the treatment of tardive dyskinesia.

H. Hemolytic And Sickle Cell Anemias

An abnormally low red blood cell (RBC) count (anemia), may be caused by a high rate of cell destruction (hemolytic anemia). Increased oxidation of cell membranes may be a factor in the mechanism of RBC lysis. Vitamin E stabilizes cell membranes. Increased RBC fragility in adults and hemolytic anemia in premature infants are symptoms of vitamin E deficiency.

Glucose-6-phosphate dehydrogenase (G6PD) deficiency is a genetic disorder that reduces RBC antioxidant capacity and survival time and therefore causes a chronic hemolytic anemia. Significantly low serum α–tocopherol levels have been reported in G6PD-deficient patients (Corash et al., 1981). The possibility that supplemental vitamin E may protect cell membranes from oxidation and consequently increase RBC lifespan has been investigated in individuals with G6PD deficiency. Administration of 800 IU/day of vitamin E over 1 year to patients with G6PD deficiency significantly improved RBC lifespan and hemoglobin concentration (Corash et al., 1980) and other hematological variables (Eldamhougy et al., 1988). Supplementation also decreased reticulocyte (immature RBC) levels, an indication of slowed RBC turnover. The same dose of vitamin E given for 2 months to children with G6PD deficiency also resulted in significant improvement in measures of RBC half-life, hemoglobin, hematocrit, and reticulocytes (Hafez et al., 1986) (Table 8).

Another genetic disorder leading to hemolysis, sickle cell anemia (SCA), causes a deformation of RBCs. Most cells are restored to the normal shape when completely oxygenated, but some remain abnormal (irreversibly sickled). A higher proportion of irreversibly to reversibly sickled cells is associated with greater cell destruction and more severe anemia (Serjeant et al., 1969; Jain, 1989). In one study a 450 IU/day vitamin E supplement given to subjects with sickle cell anemia was associated with a significant decrease in the percentage of irreversibly sickled cells (25% pretreatment

Table 8 Effect of Vitamin E Therapy[a] on Hematological Status in Patients with G6PD Deficiency

Parameter	Control (n = 14)	Treated subjects (n = 18)		P
		Before treatment	After treatment	
Hemoglobin (g/dl)				
	12.1 ± 0.9	9.0 ± 0.4	9.9 ± 0.4	<0.05
Packed cell volume (%)				
	38.1 ± 1.4	28.1 ± 1.3	30.5 ± 1.3	<0.05
Reticulocytic count (%)				
	0.71 ± 0.2	3.0 ± 0.2	2.3 ± 0.2	<0.05
Red cell half-life (days)				
	28.0 ± 0.7	16.9 ± 1.8	22.8 ± 4.6	<0.01
Serum vitamin E (mg/dl)				
	0.95 ± 0.06	0.50 ± 0.04	1.15 ± 0.13	<0.001

Values represent mean ± SEM.
[a]800 IU/day for 2 months.
Source: Adapted from Hafez et al., 1986.

to 11% posttreatment) (Natta et al., 1980). Positive results were also seen with 400 IU/day vitamin E supplementation (Jain, 1989).

In a recent study subjects with sickle cell anemia were reported to have deficient levels of vitamin E (Baliga et al., 1989). Blood from these subjects was found to form more oxygen free radicals, whereas their polymorphonuclear leukocytes (PML) had reduced capacity to generate an oxidative burst. Vitamin E supplementation increased vitamin E status and normalized these parameters. This study suggests that individuals with SCA require increased protection from free radicals. In addition, immune system impairment (in the form of reduced PML function) may be ameliorated by vitamin E supplementation in these subjects.

Although these trials are few, the results are encouraging. Further clinical investigation into a possible therapeutic benefit of vitamin E in the treatment of some of the genetic hemolytic anemias appears warranted.

IV. SAFETY

Even at very high levels of intake, vitamin E toxicity in animals is low (Bendich and Machlin, 1988). Animal studies have not indicated any carcinogenic (Wheldon et al., 1983) or teratogenic (Martin and Hurley, 1977) effect of vitamin E.

High intake of vitamin E by human subjects has generally been considered safe, with few side effects (Farrell and Bieri, 1975), although some concerns about high intravenous doses of the vitamin for premature infants have been raised (Lemons and Maisels, 1985). Reports of various side effects of vitamin E supplementation have appeared in the literature, including creatinuria and fatigue. These effects have not been seen in controlled studies. Gastric upset has been noted in some studies, but its incidence is low (Bendich and Machlin, 1988). Tsai et al. (1978) found a decrease in thyroid hormone levels following vitamin E supplementation, although no difference from controls was seen in other studies (Farrell and Bieri, 1975; Bierenbaum et al., 1985).

Vitamin E supplementation has been found to potentiate an increase in blood clotting time in individuals with disease- or drug-induced vitamin K deficiency (*Nutrition Reviews*, 1975; Corrigan, 1982). Therefore, high levels of vitamin E are not advised during anticoagulant therapy.

V. SUMMARY

Vitamin E functions in the body as the major lipid-soluble antioxidant, helping to protect the body against the injurious effects of excessive free radicals.

Generally, individuals who develop cancer have had lower blood levels of vitamin E than control subjects in prospective studies. In some, but not all, studies, the relative risk of developing cancer was higher in individuals with poorer vitamin E status.

Vitamin E decreases platelet aggregation in diabetic patients but is not very effective in normal individuals. Supplements of 200 IU/day reduced in vitro platelet activity in women on oral contraceptives and 400 IU/day inhibited in vitro platelet adhesion to collagen in healthy adults. These effects on platelet function suggest a role for vitamin E in the prevention of thrombotic disease.

Supplements of 300 IU/day appear to improve intermittent claudication.

Mortality from ischemic heart disease was inversely related to blood vitamin E levels.

Children with a high vitamin E status had improved responses in some indices of immune function. Elderly subjects with blood levels of vitamin E over 1.35 mg/dl had fewer infections than those with lower levels. Generally, an intake of 40–60 IU vitamin E per day would be needed to reach this blood level. Aministration of 800 IU/day to normal elderly subjects enhanced several parameters of immune function.

Consumption of a vitamin E supplement (usually 400 IU/day) reduced the relative risk of developing cataracts.

Heavy exercise is associated with increased lipid peroxidation, and this increase can be moderated by vitamin E supplementation. Study results suggest that vitamin E may help protect against exercise-induced muscle injury.

Administration of 1200 IU/day vitamin E resulted in significant improvement in symptoms of tardive dyskinesia.

In a limited number of trials, vitamin E supplementation appears to alleviate anemia in G6PD deficient subjects, and to reduce the proportion of irreversibly sickled RBCs in sickle cell anemia.

Vitamin E intake at high levels has been found to be safe in human and animal studies, with a low incidence of mild and reversible side effects. Vitamin E supplementation is contraindicated during anticoagulant therapy.

REFERENCES

Baker, H., Frank, O., DeAngelis, B., and Feingold, S. (1980). Plasma tocopherol in man at various times after ingesting free or acetylated tocopherol. *Nutr. Rep. Int. 21*:531–536.

Baliga, B. S., Sindel, L. J., Smith, C. J., Jenkins, L. D., Bendich, A., and Mankad, V. N. (1989). Chemiluminesence response of polymorphonuclear leukocytes from vitamin E deficient sickle cell patients. *Nutr. Rep. Int. 39*:761–771.

Bendich, A. and Machlin, L. J. (1988). Safety of oral intake of vitamin E. *Am. J. Clin. Nutr. 48*:612–619.

Bertram, J. S., Kolonel, L. N., and Meyskens, F. L., Jr. (1987). Rationale and strategies for chemoprevention of cancer in humans. *Cancer Res. 47*:3012–3031.

Bhuyan, K. C., Bhuyan, D. K., and Podos, S. M. (1982). The role of vitamin E in therapy of cataract in animals. *Ann. NY Acad. Sci. 393*:169–171.

Bierenbaum, M. L., Noonan, F. J., Machlin, L. J., Machlin, S., Stier, A., Watson, P. B., Naso, A. M., and Fleischman, A. I. (1985). The effect of supplemental vitamin E on serum parameters in diabetics, post coronary and normal subjects. *Nutr. Rep. Int. 31*:1171–1180.

Bright-See, E. and Newmark, H. L. (1983). Potential and probable role of vitamin C and E in the prevention of carcinogenesis. In *Modulation and Mediation of Cancer by Vitamins*, F. L. Meyskens and K. N. Prasad (Eds.,). Karger, New York, pp. 95–103.

Burton, K. P. (1988). Evidence of direct toxic effects of free radicals on the myocardium. *Free Radical Biol. Med. 4*:15–24.

Cadet, J. L. (1986). The potential use of vitamin E and selenium in parkinsonism. *Med. Hypothesis 20*:87–94.

Cadet, J. L., Lohr, J. B., and Jeste, D. V. (1986). Free radicals and tardive dyskinesia. *Trends Neurosci. 9*:107–108.

Calne, D. B., Eisen, A., McGeer, E., and Spencer, P. (1986). Alzheimer's disease, Parkinson's disease, and motoneurone disease: abiotropic interaction between ageing and environment? *Lancet 2*:1067–1070.

Cavarocchi, N. C., England, M. D., O'Brien, J. F., Solis, E., Russo, P., Schaff, H. V., Orszulak, T. A., Pluth, J. R., and Kaye, M. P. (1986). Superoxide generation during cardiopulmonary bypass: is there a role for vitamin E? *J. Surg. Res. 40*:519–527.

Chavance, M., Brubacher, G., Herbeth, B., Vernhes, G., Mikstacki, T., Dete, F., Fournier, C., and Janot, C. (1984). Immunological and nutritional status among the elderly. In *Lymphoid Cell Function in Aging*, A. L. deWeek (Ed.,). Eurage, Rajswik, Netherlands, pp. 231–237.

Chiu, R. C. J., Abraham, R., Mersereau, W., and Batist, G. (1987). Prefeeding of vitamin E enhances myocardial tolerance to ischemic injuries. *Clin. Invest. Med. 10*:C43.

Colette, C., Pares-Herbute, N., Monnier, L. H., and Cartry, E. (1988). Platelet function in type I diabetes: effects of supplementation with large doses of vitamin E. *Am. J. Clin. Nutr. 47*:256–261.

Colwell, J. A., Winocour, P. D., and Halushka, P. V. (1983). Do platelets have anything to do with diabetic microvascular disease? *Diabetes 32* (suppl. 2): 14–19.

Corash, L., Spielberg, S., Bartsocas, C., Boxer, L., Steinherz, R., Sheetz, M., Egan, M., Schlessleman, J., and Schulman, J. D. (1980). Reduced chronic hemolysis during high-dose vitamin E administration in Mediterranean-type glucose-6-phosphate dehydrogenase deficiency. *N. Engl. J. Med. 303*:416–420.

Corash, L., Bieri, J. G., Bashan, N., Moses, S., and Schulman, J. D. (1981). Chronic hemolysis and reduced serum alpha-tocopherol levels in glucose-6-phosphate dehydrogenase deficient Kurdish and Iraqi males. *Am. J. Clin. Nutr. 34*: 626.

Corrigan, J. J., Jr. (1982). The effect of vitamin E on warfarin–induced vitamin K deficiency. *Ann. NY Acad. Sci. 393*:361–368.

Corwin, L. M. and Gordon, R. K. (1982). Vitamin E and immune regulation. *Ann. NY Acad. Sci. 393*:437–451.

Cutler, R. G. (1976). Cross-linkage hypothesis of aging: DNA adducts in chromatin as a primary aging process. In *Aging, Carcinogenesis, and*

Radiation Biology, K. C. Smith (Ed.,). Plenum Press, New York, pp. 443–492.

Dillard, C. J., Litov, R. E., Savin, W. M., Dumelin, E. E., and Tappel, A. L. (1978). Effects of exercise, vitamin E, and ozone on pulmonary function and lipid peroxidation. *J. Appl. Physiol. 45*:927–932.

Dion, P. W., Bright-See, E. B., Smith, C. C., and Bruce, W. R. (1982). The effect of dietary ascorbic acid and alpha-tocopherol on fecal mutagenicity. *Mutation Res. 102*:27–37.

Eldamhougy, S., Elhelw, Z., Yamamah, G., Hussein, L., Fayyad, I., and Fawzy, D. (1988). The vitamin E status among glucose-6 phosphate dehydrogenase deficient patients and effeciveness of oral vitamin E. *Int. J. Vit. Nutr. Res. 58*:184–188.

Ernster, V. L., Goodson, W. H., Hunt, T. K., Petrakis, N. L., Sickles, E. A., and Miike, R. (1985). Vitamin-E and benign breast disease: a double-blind, randomized clinical trial. *Surgery 97*: 490–494.

Factor, S. A. and Weiner, W. J. (1989). Retrospective evaluation of vitamin E therapy in Parkinson's disease. *Ann. NY Acad. Sci. 570*: 441–422.

Fahn, S., (1989). The endogenous toxin hypothesis of the etiology of Parkinson's disease and a pilot trial of high-dosage antitoxidants in an attempt to slow the progression of the illness. *Ann. NY Acad. Sci. 570*: 186–196.

Farrell, P. M. (1980). Deficiency states, pharmacological effects, and nutrient requirements. In *Vitamin E: A Comprehensive Treatise*, L. J. Machlin (Ed.,). Marcel Dekker, New York, pp. 520– 620.

Farrell, P. M. and Bieri, J. G. (1975). Megavitamin E supplementation in man. *Am. J. Clin. Nutr. 28*:1381–1386.

Ferrari, R., Cargnoni, A., Ceconi, C., Curello, S., Albertini, A., and Visioli, O. (1987). Role of oxygen in the myocardial ischaemic and reperfusion damage: protective effects of vitamin E. In *Clinical and Nutritional Aspects of Vitamin E*, O. Hayaski and M. Mino (Eds.,). Elsevier Scientific Publishers, New York, pp. 209–226.

Fong, J. S. C. (1976). Alpha-tocopherol: its inhibition on human platelet aggregation. *Experientia 32*:639–641.

Gey, K. F., Brubacher, G. B., and Stahelin, H. B. (1987). Plasma levels of antioxidant vitamins in relation to ischemic heart disease and cancer. *Am. J. Clin. Nutr. 45*:1368–1377.

Gohil, K., Rothfuss, L., Lang, J., and Packer, L. (1987). Effect of exercise training on tissue vitamin E and ubiquinone content. *J. Appl. Physiol. 63*:1638–1641.

Grimes, J. D., Hassan, M. N., and Thakar, J. (1987). Antioxidant therapy in Parkinson's disease. *Can. J. Neurol. Sci. 14*:483–487.

Gwebu, E. T., Trewyn, R. W., Cornwell, D. G., and Panganamala, R. V. (1980). Vitamin E and the inhibition of platelet lipoxygenase. *Res. Commun. Chem. Pathol. Pharmacol. 28*:361–376.

Haeger, K. (1973). Walking distance and arterial flow during longterm treatment of intermittent claudication with d-alpha-tocopherol. *Vasa 2*:280–287.

Haegar, K. (1974). Long-time treatment of intermittent claudication with vitamin E. *Am. J. Clin. Nutr. 27*:1179–1181.

Haeger, K. (1978). Long-term observation of patients with atherosclerotic dysbasia on alpha-tocopherol treatment. In *Tocopherol, Oxygen and Biomembranes*, C. de Duve and O. Hayaishi (Eds.). Elsevier/North-Holland Biomedical Press, pp 329–332.

Haeger, K. (1982). Long-term study of alpha-tocopherol in intermittent claudication. *Ann. NY Acad. Sci. 393*:369–375.

Haenszel, W., Correa, P., Lopez, A., Cuello, C., Zarama, G., Zavala, D., and Fontham, E. (1985). Serum micronutrient levels in relation to gastric pathology. *Int. J. Cancer 36*:43–48.

Hafez, M., Amar, E-S., Zedan, M., Hammad, H., Sorour, A. H., El-Desouky, E-S. A., and Gamil, N. (1986). Improved erthrocyte survival with combined vitamin E and selenium therapy in children with glucose-6-phosphate dehydrogenase deficiency and mild chronic hemolysis. *J. Pediatr. 108*:558–561.

Harding, A. E., (1987). Vitamin E and the nervous system. *Crit. Rev. Neurobiol. 3*:89–103.

Harman, D. and Miller, R. W. (1986). Effect of vitamin-E on the immune response to influenza virus vaccine and the incidence of infectious disease in man. *Age 9*:21–23.

Heinonen, P. K., Koskinen, T., and Tuimala, R. (1985). Serum levels of vitamins A and E in women with ovarian cancer. *Arch. Gynecol. 237*:37–40.

Helgheim, I., Hetland, O., Nilsson, S., Ingjer, F., and Stromme, S. B. (1979). The effects of vitamin E on serum enzyme levels following heavy exercise. *Eur. J. Appl. Physiol. 40*:283–289.

Housley, E. and McFadyen, I. J. (1974). Vitamin E in intermittent claudication. *Lancet 1*:458.

Howard, L., Ovesen, L., Satya-Murti, S., and Chu, R. (1982). Reversible neurological symptoms caused by vitamin E deficiency in a patient with short bowel syndrome. *Am. J. Clin. Nutr. 36*:1243–1249.

Huijgens, P. C., van den Berg, C. A. M., Imandt, L. M. F. M., and Langenhuijsen, M. M. A. C. (1981). Vitamin E and platelet aggregation. *Acta Haematol. 65*:217–218.

Ingold, K. U., Webb, A. C., Witter, D., Burton, G. W., Metcalfe, T. A., and Muller, D. P. R. (1987). Vitamin E remains the major lipid-soluble, chain-breaking antixidant in human plasma even in individuals suffering severe vitamin E deficiency. *Arch. Biochem. Biophys.* *259*:224–225.

Ip, C. and White, G. (1987). Mammary cancer chemoprevention by inorganic and organic selenium: single agent treatment or in combination with vitamin E and their effects on in vitro immune functions. *Carcinogenesis 8*:1763–1766.

Jacques, P. F., Hartz, S. C., Chylack, L. T., Jr., McGandy, R. B., and Sadowski, J. A. (1988a). Nutritional status in persons with and without senile cataract: blood vitamin and mineral levels. *Am. J. Clin. Nutr. 48*:152–158.

Jacques, P. F., Chylack, L. T., Jr., McGandy, R. B., and Hartz, S. C. (1988b). Antioxidant status in persons with and without senile cataract. *Arch. Opthalmol. 106*:337–340.

Jain, S. K. (1989). Vitamin E and membrane abnormalaties in red cells of sickle cell disease and newborn infants. *Ann. NY Acad. Sci. 570*:461–463.

Jandak, J., Steiner, M., and Richardson, P. D. (1988). Reduction of platelet adhesiveness by vitamin E supplementation in humans. *Thrombosis Res. 49*:393–404.

Karpen, C. W., Cataland, S., O'Dorisio, T. M., and Panganamala, V. (1984). Interrelation of platelet vitamin E and thromboxane synthesis in type I diabetes mellitus. *Diabetes 33*:239–243.

Karpen, C. W., Cataland, S., O'Dorisio, T. M., and Panganamala, V. (1985). Production of 12-hydroxyeicosatetraenoic acid and vitamin E status in platelets from type I human diabetic subjects. *Diabetes 34*:526–531.

Knekt, P., Aromaa, A., Maatela, J., Aaran, R. K., Nikkari, T., Hakama, M., Hakulinen, T., Peto, R., Saxen, E., and Teppo, L. (1988). Serum vitamin E and risk of cancer among Finnish men during a 10-year follow-up. *Am. J. Epidemiol. 127*:28–41.

Kok, F. J., van Duijn, C. M., Hofman, A., Vermeeren, R., de Bruijn, A. M., and Valkenburg, H. A. (1987). Micronutrients and the risk of lung cancer. *N. Engl. J. Med. 316*:1416.

Lafuze, J. E., Weisman, S. J., Alperty, L. A., and Baehner, R. L. (1984). Vitamin E attenuates the effects of FMLP on rabbit circulating granulocytes. *Pediatr. Res. 18*:536–540.

Lawrence, L. M., Mathias, M. M., Nockels, C. F., and Tengerdy, R. P. (1985). The effect of vitamin E on prostaglandin levels in the immune organs of chicks during the course of an *E. coli* infection. *Nutr. Res. 5*:497–509.

Lehmann, J., Rao, D. D., Canary, J. J., and Judd, J. T. (1988). Vitamin E and relationships among tocopherols in human plasma, platelets, lymphocytes, and red blood cells. *Am. J. Clin. Nutr. 47*:470–474.

Lemons, J. A. and Maisels, M. J. (1985). Vitamin E—how much is too much? *Pediatrics* 76:625–627.

Lemoyne, M., Van Gossum, A., Kurian, R. T., Ostro, M., Axler, J., and Jeejeebhoy, K. N. (1987). Breath pentane analysis as an index of lipid peroxidation: a functional test of vitamin E status. *Am. J. Clin. Nutr.* 46:267–272.

Likoff, R. O., Guptill, D. R., Lawrence, L. M., McKay, C. C., Mathias, M. M., Nockels, C. F., and Tenderdy, R. P. (1981). Vitamin E and aspirin depress prostaglandins in protection of chickens against *Escherichia coli* infection. *Am. J. Clin. Nutr.* 34:245–251.

Lohr, J. B., Cadet, J. L., Lohr, M. A., Jeste, D. V., and Wyatt, R. J. (1987). Alpha-tocopherol in tardive dyskinesia. *Lancet 1*:913.

London, R. S., Murphy, L., and Kitlowski, K. E. (1985a). Hypothesis: Breast cancer prevention by supplemental vitamin E. *J. Am. Coll. Nutr. 4*:559–564.

London, R. S., Sundaram, G. S., Murphy, L., Manimekalai, S., Reynolds, M., and Goldstein, P. J. (1985b). The effect of vitamin E on mammary dysplasia: a double-blind study. *Obstet. Gynecol. 65*:104–106.

Martin, M. M. and Hurley, L. S. (1977). Effect of large amounts of vitamin E during pregnancy and lactation. *Am. J. Clin. Nutr. 30*:1629–1637.

Massey, K. D., Pasteur, W. E., and Burton, K. P. (1986). Administration of alpha-tocopherol preserves myocardial membrane integrity during ischemia and reperfusion. *Circulation 74*:434.

McCord, J. M. (1985). Oxygen-derived free radicals in postischemic tissue injury. *N. Engl. J. Med. 312*:159–163.

McCord, J. M. (1988). Free radicals and myocardial ischemia: overview and outlook. *Free Radical Biol. Med. 4*:9–14.

Meeker, H. C., Eskew, M. L., Scheuchenzuber, W., Scholz, R. W., and Zarkower, A. (1985). Antioxidant effects on cell-mediated immunity. *J. Leukocyte Biol.38*:451–458.

Menkes, M. S., Comstock, G. W., Vuilleumier, J. P., Helsing, K. J., Rider, A. A., and Brookmeyer, R. (1986). Serum beta-carotene vitamins A and E, selenium, and the risk of lung cancer. *N. Engl. J. Med. 315*:1250–1254.

Mergens, W. J., Kamm, J. J., and Newmark, H. L. (1978). Alpha-tocopherol: uses in preventing nitrosamine formation. In *Environmental Aspects of N-Nitroso Compounds*, E. A. Walker, M. Castegnaro, L. Griciute, and R. E. Lyle, (Eds.,). IARC Scientific Publications, Lyon, pp. 19–212.

Meydani, S. N., Barklund, M. P., Liu, S., Meydani, M., Miller, R., Cannon, J., Morrow, F., Rocklin, R., and Blumberg, J. (1989). Effect of vitamin E supplementation on immune responsiveness of healthy elderly subjects. *FASEB J. 3*:A1057.

Mirvish, S. S. (1986). Effects of vitamins C and E on *N*-nitroso compound formation, carcinogenesis, and cancer. *Cancer 58*: 1842–1850.

Miyamoto, H., Araya, Y., Ito, M., Hiroshi, I., Dosaka, H., Shimizu, T., Kishi, F., Yamamoto, I., Honma, H., and Kawakami, Y. (1987). Serum selenium and vitamin E concentrations in families of lung cancer patients. *Cancer 60*:1159–1162.

Muller, D. P. R. (1986). Vitamin E—its role in neurological function. *Postgrad. Med. J. 62*:107–112.

Muller, D. P. R., Lloyd, J. K., and Wolff, O. H. (1983). Vitamin E and neurological function. *Lancet 1*:225–228.

Natta, C. L., Machlin, L. J., and Brin, M. (1980). A decrease in irreversibly sickled erthrocytes in sickle cell anemia patients given vitamin E. *Am. J. Clin. Nutr. 33*:968–971.

Newmark, H. L. and Mergens, W. J. (1981). Alpha-Tocopherol (vitamin E) and its relationship to tumor induction and development. In *Inhibition of Tumor Induction and Development*, M. S. Zedeck and M. Lipkin, (Eds.,). Plenum Press, New York, pp. 127–168.

Nomura, A. M. Y., Stemmermann, G. N., Heilbrun, L. K., Salkeld, R. M., and Vuilleumier, J. P. (1985). Serum vitamin levels and the risk of cancer of specific sites in men of Japanese ancestry in Hawaii. *Cancer Res. 45*:2369–2372.

Nutrition Reviews 1975. Hypervitaminosis E and coagulation. *Nutr. Rev. 33*:269–270.

Oshima, H. and Bartsch, H. (1981). Quantitative estimation of endogenous nitrosation in humans by monitoring *N*-nitrosoproline excreted in the urine. *Cancer Res. 41*:3658–3662.

Packer, L. (1984). Vitamin E, physical exercise and tissue damage in animals. *Med. Biol. 62*:105–109.

Petersen, H. D. and Gormsen, J. (1978). Platelet aggregation in diabetes mellitus. *Acta Med. Scand. 203*:125–130.

Pincemail, J., Deby, C., Dethier, A., Bertrand, Y., Lismonde, M., and Lamy, M. (1987). Pentane measurement in man as an index of lipoperoxidation. *J. Electroanal. Chem. 232*:117–125.

Pincemail, J., Deby, C., Camus, G., Pirnay, F., Bouchez, R., Massaux, L., and Goutier, R. (1988). Tocopherol mobilization during intensive exercise. *Eur. J. Appl. Physiol. 57*:189–191.

Pinsky, M. J. (1980). Treatment of intermittent claudication with alpha-tocopherol. *J. Am. Podiatry Assoc. 70*:454–458.

Prasad, J. S. (1980). Effect of vitamin E supplementation on leukocyte function. *Am. J. Clin. Nutr. 33*:606–608.

Quintanilha, A. T. (1984). Effects of physical exercise and/or vitamin E on tissue oxidative metabolism. *Biochem. Soc. Trans. 12*:403–404.

Renaud, S., Ciavatti, M., Perrot, L., Berthezene, F., Dargent, D., and Condamin, P. (1987). Influence of vitamin E administration on platelet functions in hormonal contraceptive users. *Contraception 36*:347–358.

Robertson, J. M., Donner, A. P., and Trevithick, J. R. (1989). Vitamin E intake and risk of cataract in humans. *Ann. NY Acad. Sci. 570*:372–382.

Russ, H., Mihatsch, W., Kuhn, W., and Przuntek, H. (1987). MPTP model of Parkinson's disease in marmoset: radical scavengers do not prevent neurodegeneration. *J. Neurochem. 48*(suppl.):S159.

Russell, M. J., Thomas, B. S., and Bulbrook, R. D. (1988). A prospective study of the relationship between serum vitamins A and E and risk of breast cancer. *Br. J. Cancer 57*:213–215.

Salonen, J. T., Salonen, R., Lappetelainen, R., Maenpaa, P. H., Alfthan, G., and Puska, P. (1985). Risk of cancer in relation to serum concentrations of selenium and vitamins A and E: matched case-control analysis of prospective data. *Br. Med. J. 290*:417–420.

Sergeant, G. R., Serjeant, B. E., and Milner, P. F. (1969). The irreversibly sickled cell; a determinant of haemolysis in sickle cell anemia. *Br. J. Haematol. 17*:527–533.

Shklar, G. and Schwartz, J. (1988). Tumor necrosis factor in experimental cancer regression with vitamin E, beta carotene, canthaxanthin and algae extract. *Eur. J. Cancer Clin. Oncol. 24*:839–850.

Shklar, G., Schwartz, J., Trickler, D. P., and Niukian, K. (1987). Regression by vitamin E of experimental oral cancer. *J. Natl. Cancer Inst. 78*:987–992.

Simon-Schnass, I., Pabst, H., and Herrligkoffer, K. M. (1987). [Effect of vitamin E on exercise parameters in high altitude mountaineering] [Ger]. *Deutsch Z. Sportmedi. 38*:200–206.

Sokol, R. J. (1989). Vitamin E and neurologic function in man. *Free Rad. Biol. Med. 6*:189–207.

Stahelin, H. B., Rosel,F., Buess, E., and Brubacher, G. (1984). Cancer, vitamins, and plasma lipids: prospective Basel study. *J. Natl. Cancer Inst. 73*:1463–1468.

Stampfer, M. J., Jakubowski, J. A., Faigel, D., Vaillancourt, R., and Deykin, D. (1988). Vitamin E supplementation effect on human platelet function, arachidonic acid metabolism, and plasma prostacyclin levels. *Am. J. Clin. Nutr. 47*:700–706.

Steiner, M. (1981). Vitamin E changes the membrane fluidity of human platelets. *Biochim. Biophys. Acta 640*:100–105.

Steiner, M. (1983). Effect of alpha-tocopherol administration on platelet function in man. *Thromb. Haemostas. 49*:73–77.

Steiner, M. (1987). Effect of vitamin E on platelet function and thrombosis. *Agents Actions 22*:357–358.

Steiner, M. and Anastasi, J. (1976). Vitamin E: an inhibitor of the platelet release reaction. *J. Clin. Invest. 57*:732–737.

Steiner, M. and Mower, R. (1982). Mechanism of action of vitamin E on platelet function. *Ann. NY Acad. Sci. 393*:289–299.

Sundaram, G. S., London, R., Manimekalai, S., Nair, P. P., and Goldstein, P. (1981). Alpha-tocopherol and serum lipoproteins. *Lipids 16*:223–227.

Szczeklik, A., Gryglewski, R. J., Domagala, B., Dworski, R., and Basista, M. (1985). Dietary supplementation with vitamin E in hyperlipoproteinemias: effects on plasma lipid peroxides, antioxidant activity, prostacyclin generation and platelet aggregability. *Thromb. Haemostas. 54*:425–430.

Tappel, A. L. (1973). Lipid peroxidation damage to cell components. *Fed. Proc. 32*:1870–1874.

Tappel, A. L. (1974). Selenium-gluthathione peroxidase and vitamin E. *Am. J. Clin. Nutr. 27*:960–965.

Tappel, A. L. and Dillard, C. J. (1981). In vivo lipid peroxidation: measurement via exhaled pentane and protection by vitamin E. *Fed. Proc. 40*:174–178.

Taylor, A. (1989). Associations between nutrition and cataract. *Nutr. Rev. 47*:225–234.

Tengerdy, R. P. (1980). Effect of vitamin E on immune responses. In: *Vitamin E: A Comprehensive Treatise*, L. J. Machlin (Ed.,). Marcel Dekker, New York, pp. 429–444.

Tsai, A. C., Kelley, J. J., Peng, B., and Cook, N. (1978). Study on the effect of megavitamin E supplementation in man. *Am. J. Clin. Nutr. 31*:831–837.

Tuyns, A. J., Riboli, E., and Doornbos, G. (1985). Nutrition and cancer of the esophagus. In *Diet and Human Carcinogenesis*, J. V. Joossens, et al. (Eds.,). Elsevier Science Publishers, New York, pp. 71–79.

Varma, S. D., Chand, D., Sharma, Y. R., Kuck, J. F., and Richards, R. D. (1984). Oxidative stress on lens and cataract formation: role of light and oxygen. *Curr. Eye Res. 3*:35–57.

Vatassery, G. T., Johnson, G. J., and Krezowski, A. M. (1983). Changes in vitamin E concentrations in human plasma and platelets with age. *J. Am. Coll. Nutr. 4*:369–375.

Vericel, E., Croset, M., Sedivy, P., Courpron, P., Dechavanne, M., and Lagarde, M. (1988). Platelets and aging, I. Aggregation, arachidonate metabolism and antioxidant status. *Thrombosis Res. 49*:331–342.

Vobecky, J. S., Vobecky, J., and Rola-Pleszczynski, M. (1986a). The comparison between immune status and nutrient intake in preschoolers. In *Recent Advances in Clinical Nutrition: 2*, M. L. Wahlqvist and A. S. Truswell (Eds.,). John Libbey, London, pp. 372–376.

Vobecky, J. S., Vobecky, J., Shapcott, D., and Rola-Pleszczynski, M.(1986b). Humoral and cell-mediated immunity in relation to the serum level of selected nutrients in pre-schoolers. In: *Recent Advances in Clinical Nutrition: 2*, M. L. Wahlqvist and A. S. Truswell (Eds.,). John Libbey, London, pp. 369–372.

Vorherr, H. (1986). Fibrocystic breast disease: pathophysiology, pathomorphology, clinical picture, and management. *Am. J. Obstet. Gynecol. 154*:161–179.

Wald, N. J., Boreham, J., Hayward, J. L., and Bulbrook, R. D. (1984). Plasma retinol, beta-carotene and vitamin E levels in relation to the future risk of breast cancer. *Br. J. Cancer 49*:321–324.

Wald, N. J., Thompson, S. G., Densem, J. W., Boreham, J., and Bailey, A. (1987). Serum vitamin E and subsequent risk of cancer. *Br. J. Cancer 56*:69–72.

Wald, N. J., Nicolaides-Bouman, A., and Hudson, G. A. (1988). Plasma retinol, beta-carotene and vitamin E levels in relation to the future risk of breast cancer. *Br. J. Cancer 57*:235.

Watanabe, J., Umeda, F., Wakasugi, H., and Ibayaski, H. (1984). Effect of vitamin E on platelet aggregation in diabetes mellitus. *Thromb. Haemostas. 51*:313–316.

Wheldon, G. H., Bhatt, A., Keller, P., and Hummler, H. (1983). d, l-Alpha-tocopherol acetate (vitamin E): a long term toxicity and carcinogenicity study in rats. *Int. J. Vit. Nutr. Res. 53*:287–296.

Willett, W. C., Polk, B. F., Underwood, B. A., Stampfer, M. J., Pressel, S., Rosner, B., Taylor, J. O., Schneider, K., and Hames, C. G. (1984). Relation of serum vitamins A and E and carotenoids to the risk of cancer. *N. Engl. J. Med. 310*:430–434.

Williams, H. T. G., Fenna, D., and Macbeth, R. A. (1971). Alpha tocopherol in the treatment of intermittent claudication. *Surg. Gynecol. Obstet. 132*:662–666.

6

Vitamin C

S. K. Gaby and V. N. Singh

I. INTRODUCTION

Vitamin C (ascorbic acid and dehydroascorbic acid) is a water-soluble essential nutrient for humans and other primates, the Indian fruit bat, guinea pigs, and most fish. Good dietary sources of vitamin C include citrus and other fruits, cruciferous vegetables, peppers, and potatoes.

The deficiency disease associated with vitamin C is scurvy. The symptoms of scurvy include fatigue, joint and muscle pain, skin lesions, gum disease, and generalized capillary bleeding.

A. Metabolism and Function

Vitamin C is required for the conversion of tyrosine to dopamine and other neurotransmitters, and may be involved in steroid synthesis and microsomal drug metabolism (Table 1).

Ascorbic acid is also necessary for collagen metabolism. Collagen is the most common protein in the body and a component of the supporting structures of skin, cartilage, tendons, ligaments, bones, teeth, and blood vessels. After collagen protein is synthesized, its proline and lysine amino acid residues undergo hydroxylation, allowing the molecule to attain its optimal configuration. Vitamin C is required for the hydroxylation step, without

103

which the collagen is weak and easily damaged. This poorly formed collagen appears to be more susceptible to collagenolytic (breakdown) enzymes (Schneir et al., 1985). In addition, recent in vitro work suggests that ascorbic acid acts directly to increase procollagen messenger RNA levels in human fibroblasts (Geesin et al., 1988). Collagen subunits are formed within fibroblasts as procollagen, which is excreted into extracellular spaces. Vitamin C is required to export the procollagen molecules out of the cell. The final (quartenary) structure of the collagen is formed after pieces of the procollagen are enzymatically cleaved.

Ascorbic acid is an antioxidant (Bendich et al., 1986; see Introduction). Vitamin C has been shown to scavenge peroxyl radicals (Niki et al., 1983), superoxide radicals (Som et al., 1983), and myeloperoxidase–derived hypochlorous acid (Halliwell et al., 1987). In human plasma, ascorbate is the only antioxidant capable of protecting lipids from aqueous peroxyl radical-induced oxidative damage, trapping essentially all aqueous peroxyl.

B. Absorption and Requirements

An adult requires 10 mg/day of dietary ascorbic acid to prevent scurvy. The U.S. Recommended Daily Allowance (RDA) for vitamin C is 60 mg/day, however, tissue saturation appears to require an ascorbic acid intake in excess of 100 mg/day (Schorah, 1978). A daily intake of 100 mg of vitamin C

Table 1   Major Biochemical Functions Requiring Vitamin C

Collagen metabolism
    Stimulation of procollagen mRNA production (?)
    Hydroxylation of proline and lysine
        in collagen synthesis
    Export of collagen out of the cell
    Control of collagenolytic activity

Carnitine biosynthesis

Catecholamine biosynthesis, tyrosine metabolism

Iron metabolism absorption and mobilization
    (Reducing and chelating properties)

Histamine catabolism

Antioxidant function

Immune functions

---

is also the amount estimated to be necessary for 95% of a population of healthy, nonsmoking adult men to maintain a body pool of the vitamin of 20 mg/kg body weight (Kallner et al., 1979). Jacob et al. (1987a) conducted a well–controlled study of men consuming 5 – 605 mg of vitamin C per day. They found that 138 mg vitamin C per day maximized the body pool in healthy young men and that a marginal plasma ascorbic acid level (0.4 mg/dl) was maintained by an intake of 41 mg/day (Jacob et al., 1987a). It must be emphasized that the above requirements are meant for normal nonsmoking adults. However, as discussed below, some groups of people may need higher intakes of vitamin C.

Because of the individual variation in absorption and/or metabolism (Yew, 1975; Basu and Schorah, 1982), the range of serum levels of ascorbic acid associated with a given level of intake is quite broad. For example, a summary of a large number of published studies showed that in 95% of the population, the plasma levels of the vitamin associated with a 60 mg/day intake of ascorbic acid would range from about 0.4 mg/dl to nearly 1.0 mg/dl (Basu and Schorah, 1982).

In species requiring a dietary source of vitamin C, absorption of the nutrient is an energy-requiring, active transport process (Stevenson, 1974). The absorption mechanism in the gut and the reabsorption capacity of the kidneys are saturable. Consequently, efficient absorption of ascorbic acid (about 80% in a single bolus up to 180 mg) declines in a dose-related manner (Melethil et al., 1986). More efficient absorption is achieved through small multiple doses.

C. Risk of Inadequate Ascorbic Acid Status

Large subgroups of the U.S. population are at risk of having a poor vitamin C status.

1. Elderly

The elderly, because of poor diet, dental problems, lack of mobility, drug/nutrient interactions, and economic restraints, often suffer from inadequate nutrition. It has been suggested that there may be many cases of unrecognized scurvy, particularly among the elderly (Connelly et al., 1982). A comparison of mean plasma vitamin C levels in young adults and elderly subjects showed that the older group had less than half the concentration of ascorbic acid found in the younger group (Schorah, 1978).

Poor ascorbic acid status in the elderly has been generally attributed to low intake (Newton et al., 1985). However, while a 1 g/day supplement of vitamin C improved ascorbic acid status in a group of elderly patients, it failed to bring plasma values up to those normally found in younger adults (Schorah et al., 1979). Institutionalized elderly subjects had a mean plasma level of the vitamin which was less than one fifth of that seen in young adults (Schorah, 1978). The range of plasma vitamin C values found in the latter group overlapped that of a group of frankly scorbutic subjects. Plasma levels of ascorbic acid were measured in healthy individuals over 65 years of age given various amounts of vitamin C (30–280 mg/day) (VanderJagt et al., 1987). The daily intakes of vitamin C required to maintain a plasma level of 1.0 mg/dl were about 150 mg for men and 80 mg for women. Vitamin C consumption at 60 mg/day (U.S. RDA) was associated with plasma ascorbic acid levels at or below 0.4 mg/dl in most of the men; this level is generally considered the lower limit of normal (VanderJagt et al., 1987). Garry et al., found similar results in healthy people over 60: women required 75 mg/day and men required 150 mg/day to maintain an ascorbic acid plasma level of 1.0 mg/dl (1982).

2. Smokers

There are over 50 million smokers in the United States. Cigarette smoking is associated with a significant decrease in ascorbic acid status (Hoefel, 1983; Keith and Mossholder, 1986). On average, smoking more than a pack a day is associated with serum vitamin C levels up to 40% lower than those of nonsmokers (Pelletier, 1977). The lower level does not appear to be the result of a simple difference in ascorbic acid intake, since an evaluation of the second National Health and Nutrition Examination Survey (NHANES II) data indicates that at a comparable intake level, smokers had a substantially lower serum vitamin C concentration than nonsmokers (Smith and Hodges, 1987; Schectman et al., 1989). These data imply that in order for smokers to achieve serum levels of the vitamin equivalent to those of nonsmokers, smokers require an additional 65.4 mg of vitamin C per day (Smith and Hodges, 1987). Similarly, Kallner et al. (1981) found a higher metabolic turnover and lower absorption of the vitamin in smokers than nonsmokers and recommended a daily intake of 140 mg to compensate for the difference and maintain a replete body pool. Recommended dietary intakes of vitamin C are higher for smokers than for nonsmokers in the United States, Canada, New Zealand, and France.

3. Alcoholics

Generally due to their poor diet, many alcoholics have a low ascorbic acid status (Bonjour, 1979), and are at risk of subclinical ascorbic acid deficiency (O'Keane et al., 1972) or scurvy, in addition to other nutritional inadequacies. Vitamin C deficiency is common among patients with alcoholic liver disease (Majumdar et al., 1983). In addition, acute ingestion of alcohol is associated with increased urinary excretion of vitamin C (Faizallah et al., 1986) and depressed plasma ascorbic acid concentrations (Fazio et al., 1981). High–dose ascorbic acid therapy (500–1000 mg/day) has been recommended in the treatment of chronic alcoholics (Piatkowski et al., 1986).

4. Diabetics

Glucose and ascorbic acid have very similar structures and are thought to share a cellular transport mechanism. Because diabetics typically have high blood glucose (hyperglycemia), the competition between glucose and vitamin C for transport into cells is likely to cause vitamin C inadequacy in tissues and organs (Ginter and Chorvathova, 1983). This cellular vitamin C inadequacy may not be associated with a lowered plasma level of vitamin C. In cells requiring insulin for glucose uptake, inadequate insulin would also result in impaired ascorbic acid transport (Mann, 1974).

Ascorbic acid levels have been reported to be low in the plasma (Stankova et al., 1984), red blood cells (Bryszewska and Kostrzewa, 1987), and white blood cells (Pecoraro and Chen, 1987) of diabetic subjects. The low plasma and tissue levels of vitamin C in rats with streptozotocin–induced diabetes were normalized by vitamin C supplementation (McLennan et al., 1988). In these animals, supplemental vitamin C also prevented a decline in the activity of an ascorbic acid-dependent enzyme involved in collagen maintenance (McLennan et al., 1988). Rats with experimentally-induced diabetes have substantially reduced new collagen production, reduced collagen hydroxylation, and increased intracellular procollagen degradation compared to normal rats; dietary vitamin C supplementation completely prevented the reduced hydroxylation and partially prevented the other changes (Schneir et al., 1985).

In a fasting state, diabetics have been reported to have a significantly lower leukocyte ascorbic acid level than normal controls (Chen et al., 1983), although this was not found in a group of diabetics in England (Schorah et al., 1988). Intravenous infusion of glucose to cause hyperglycemia in normal subjects correlated negatively with leukocyte ascorbic acid (Chen et al., 1983; Pecoraro and Chen, 1987). Prolonged experimental hyperglycemia resulted in an impairment of mononuclear and polymorphonuclear (PMN) leukocyte chemotaxis (part of the immune response) that correlated with decreases in leukocyte ascorbic acid (Pecoraro and Chen, 1987). The rate of PMN and mononuclear leukocyte dehydroascorbic acid uptake is slower in diabetic than in nondiabetic subjects (Stankova et al., 1984).

These studies indicate that the requirement for vitamin C may be higher in people with diabetes than in normal subjects. It has been suggested that vitamin C supplementation may be useful in countering some of the health problems secondary to diabetes (Ginter and Chorvathova, 1983).

5. Workers Occupationally Exposed to Pollutants

Low serum levels of vitamin C have been reported in individuals who are exposed to certain toxins in the workplace. Dawson et al., found reduced blood levels of ascorbic acid in men occupationally exposed to lead at work, in comparison with workers in other environments (1988). Coal tar workers were found to have very low serum levels of ascorbic acid, bordering on the range associated with scurvy (Sram et al., 1983a). The mean levels were lower in the coal tar workers who smoked than in those who did not (Sram et al., 1983a). The damaging effects of these low vitamin C levels are discussed below.

II. HEALTH BENEFITS

Antioxidants may play an important role in the prevention of tissue damage and disease (see Introduction). The levels of total and oxidized ascorbic acid are reduced with increasing age, suggesting a possible reduction in antioxidant status in the elderly (Sasaki et al., 1983). Evidence in support of this is the finding that supplementation with 400 mg vitamin C per day for 1 year decreased the serum lipid peroxide levels of elderly subjects (Wartanowicz et al., 1984). Increased lipid peroxidation has been associated with accelerated aging and degeneration (Tappel, 1973). The health implication of these findings remains to be established.

The antioxidant function of vitamin C may be one of the mechanisms by which the vitamin could protect DNA from free radical damage and mutagens. Ascorbic acid has been shown to reduce some potentially harmful genetic alterations, sister-chromatid exchanges, in vitro (Weitberg and Weitzman, 1985). Ascorbic acid also appears to reduce the toxic, mutagenic, and/or carcinogenic effects of many environmental pollutants, including pesticides, heavy metals, industrial–use hydrocarbons, ozone, and carbon monoxide (Calabrese, 1985). Vitamin C may exert its protection against environmental pollutants through stimulation of liver detoxifying enzymes. For this reason vitamin C has been suggested as a treatment for certain acute intoxications (Schvartsman, 1983). Chromosome aberrations in lymphocytes were significantly reduced (by about 65%) with high doses of vitamin C in coal-tar workers, whose average plasma levels of ascorbic acid rose from 0.21 mg/dl (a borderline scorbutic level) to 1.31 mg/dl after 3 months of supplements (Sram et al., 1983a). A similar effect was found in workers exposed to styrene, methyl methacrylate (Sram et al., 1986), and halogenated ethers (Sram et al., 1983b). The prophylactic effect of vitamin C appears to be most significant in individuals with a high initial concentration of aberrant cells (Sram et al., 1986). In addition, markedly low serum vitamin C levels in workers at lead smelting plants have been associated with sperm abnormalities (Dawson et al., 1988). Such abnormalities have been partially corrected by vitamin C supplementation (Dawson et al., 1987). However, vitamin C supplementation does not appear to be protective against chromosome aberrations in workers exposed to cancer chemotherapeutic agents (Rossner et al., 1988).

It has been hypothesized that vitamin C may impact human disease, specifically cancer, through the inhibition of nitrosamine formation in addition to acting as an antioxidant and stimulating liver enzymes. In human studies, oral doses of ascorbic acid significantly reduced urinary levels of nitrosamines when the precursor of a noncarcinogenic nitrosamine was consumed, but the vitamin does not appear to decrease normal or "background" nitrosamine levels in adults (Wagner et al., 1983, 1985; Garland et al., 1986; Leaf et al., 1987), including smokers (Hoffmann and Brunnemann, 1983). Vitamin C supplementation has been shown to decrease the mutagenicity of gastric juice (O'Connor et al., 1985). Vitamin C may therefore be helpful in reducing the nitrosation of abnormally high levels of environmentally introduced nitrosamine precursors (Bellander et al., 1988).

A. Vitamin C and Cancer

1. Mechanisms

It has been suggested that vitamin C may be useful in the prevention of cancer (Block and Menkes, 1989). Possible mechanisms by which vitamin C may affect carcinogenesis include: acting as an antioxidant, blocking formation of nitrosamines and fecal mutagens, enhancing immune system response (Glatthaar et al., 1986), and accelerating detoxifying liver enzymes (Newberne and Suphakarn, 1984) (see Table 2).

2. Ascorbic Acid Status of Subjects with Cancer

Evidence for the efficacy of vitamin C in the treatment of human cancer is based in part on studies showing significantly reduced levels of the vitamin in patients with malignant conditions (Greco et al., 1982; Ghosh and Das; 1985; Romney et al., 1985). Large doses of vitamin C (2–5 g/day) have been shown to correct these low serum levels and may improve immune system defenses in some such patients (Greco et al., 1982; Sergeev, 1984).

3. Cancer Treatment

Cameron and Pauling (1978) reported a significant increase over controls in survival time of cancer patients described as "terminal" and "untreatable" who received ascorbate supplementation of about 10 g/day. However, no effect on advanced cancer was seen in a placebo-controlled

Table 2   Possible Mechanisms Of Action Of Vitamin C In Reducing Cancer Risk

---

Vitamin C may protect against cancer by:
  Acting as an antioxidant
  Enhancing immune system functions
  Blocking nitrosation
  Enhancing hepatic clearance of toxins (via cytochrome P– 450)
  Blocking the formation of fecal mutagens

---

study using a 10 g/day vitamin C supplement (Moertel et al, 1985), although this study may be criticized for its short duration, inadequate checks on compliance, and evidence of possible self-supplementation by control subjects. Other investigators found no difference in survival between ascorbic acid supplemented (3 g/day) and unsupplemented groups of women with early breast cancer (Poulter et al., 1984).

Current evidence suggests that the major benefit of ascorbic acid with regard to cancer may be in reducing the risk of developing cancer, rather than in therapy.

4.   Cancer Risk Reduction

Although epidemiologists attempt to account for as many variables as possible, it is often difficult to make definite conclusions about the relationship between a specific nutrient (which is present as a component of a complex food item) and cancer. Several epidemiological studies have reported an association between a high consumption of foods rich in vitamin C and a reduced risk of certain cancers (Table 3). However, the issue is clouded by the tendency for foods rich in vitamin C to contain, simultaneously, a rich supply of certain other nutrients such as folate and β–carotene, as well as fiber.

5.   Esophageal Cancer

In case-control studies, high dietary vitamin C has been found to be associated with a lowered incidence of esophageal cancer (Cook-Mozaffari et al., 1979; Ziegler et al., 1981; Mettlin et al., 1981). A comparison of the diets of people in areas of Iran with high or low incidence of esophageal cancer showed a significantly lower intake of vitamin C and infrequent fresh vegetable and fruit consumption among people in the areas with a high incidence of the disease (Hormozdiari et al., 1975; Joint Iran–International Agency for Research, 1977).

A group at high risk for esophageal cancer in China has been reported to have a significantly higher excretion of urinary nitrosamines (Lu et al., 1986), following exposure to a noncarcinogenic precursor as compared to a group at low risk for the cancer. The food and water normally consumed by residents of the high–risk area are high in precursors of (carcinogenic) nitrosamines. The urinary nitrosamine concentration in the high–risk group was reduced to the low–risk control levels with doses of 100 mg of ascorbic acid for 3 days.

These clinical and epidemiological data suggest a possible role for dietary ascorbic acid in reducing the risk of esophageal cancer.

6. Atrophic Gastritis and Stomach Cancer

It has been proposed that stomach cancer is the end result of a long-term, progressive assault on the gastric mucosa, and that conditions such as ulcers, hypochlorhydria (inadequate hydrochloric acid production), and atrophic gastritis represent early stages in this progression (Correa et al., 1975; Correa, 1985). The formation of nitrosamines is also implicated as a factor in this model of gastric cancer development.

Studies have shown that supplements of vitamin C (1 g/day) significantly reduce both N–nitroso compound formation in cases of hypochlorhydria (Reed et al., 1983) and the mutagenicity of gastric juice from duodenal ulcer patients (O'Connor et al., 1985) (Table 4). The critical factor in reducing gastric juice mutagenic activity in the latter study was the concentration of ascorbic acid, even though there was no significant change in gastric pH (O'Connor et al., 1985). Ascorbic acid appears to have an antimutagenic effect in gastric juice only when it is present at the same time as nitrite (Norkus and Kuenzig, 1985).

Epidemiological evidence points to an inverse relationship between consumption of fruits (especially citrus, which are rich in vitamin C) and/or dietary ascorbic acid intake and the risk of developing atrophic gastritis (Fontham et al., 1986) and stomach cancer (Risch et al., 1985; Correa et al., 1985; La Vecchia et al., 1987; You et al., 1988). One study measured the plasma levels of ascorbic acid in subjects from two towns in Britain with high and low stomach cancer death rates (Burr et al., 1987). Plasma ascorbate was not related to atrophic gastritis incidence, but both plasma ascorbate and fruit intake were lower in the high-risk area.

7. Colon and Rectal Cancers

A large-scale study of dietary and other risk factors for colorectal cancer was conducted in Australia, a country with a high incidence of this disease (Kune et al., 1987). The study was designed to reflect food consumption patterns for the previous 20 years. The researchers found that dietary vitamin C was protective against colorectal cancer at intakes above 230 mg/

Table 3 Epidemiological Studies: Vitamin C And Cancer Risk

Site	Subjects	Findings	Reference
Oral/ Pharyngeal	227 cases 405 controls	Reduced risk with more frequent fruit and vegetable intake	Winn et al., 1984
Oral/ Pharyngeal	871 cases 979 controls	Reduced risk with increased fruit intake, vitamin C intake	McLaughlin et al., 1988
Oral	425 cases 588 controls	Reduced risk (dose-response) as vitamin C intake increased	Marshall et al., 1982
Pharyngeal	166 cases 547 controls	Reduced risk with increased vitamin C intake	Rossing et al., 1989
Larynx	374 cases 381 controls	Reduced risk with increased vitamin C intake	Graham et al., 1981
Esophagus	344 cases 688 controls	Reduced risk with increased intake of fresh fruit and raw vegetables	Cook-Mozaffari et al., 1979
Esophagus	120 cases 250 controls	Reduced risk with increased intake of vitamin C-rich foods	Ziegler et al., 1981
Esophagus	147 cases 264 controls	Reduced risk (dose-response) with increased ingestion of foods containing vitamin C	Mettlin et al., 1981
Esophagus	743 cases 1975 controls	Reduced risk with increased vitamin C and citrus fruit intake	Tuyns et al., 1987
Stomach	228 cases 1394 controls	Reduced risk associated with high vitamin C intake in people < 60 years old	Bjelke, 1974
Stomach	391 cases 391 controls	Reduced risk with increased fruit and dietary vitamin C.	Correa et al., 1985

Site	Cases/Controls	Finding	Reference
Stomach	246 cases 246 controls	Reduced risk with increased citrus fruit but total vitamin C intake less protective	Risch et al., 1985
Stomach	110 cases 100 cases	Reduced risk with increased lemon and orange consumption	Trichopoulos et al., 1985
Stomach	206 cases 474 controls	Reduced risk with increased fresh fruit, specifically citrus	LaVecchia et al., 1987
Stomach	564 cases 1131 controls	Reduced risk associated with greater dietary intake of vitamin C	You et al., 1988
Stomach	267 men from low- and 246 from high-risk towns	Plasma ascorbate and fruit intake were lower in the high-risk area but no direct relationship between ascorbate and atrophic gastritis	Burr et al., 1987
Stomach	188 cases 800 controls	No difference between cases and controls in frequency of citrus fruits/juice consumption	Graham et al., 1967
Bladder	164 cases 314 controls	Reduced risk with increased vitamin C intake in most groups	Kolonel et al., 1985
Cervix[a]	32 cases 71 controls	Reduced risk with vitamin C intake above the median (76 mg/day)	Wasserheil-Smoller et al. 1981
Cervix[a]	17 cases 34 controls	Reduced risk with increased serum ascorbate levels	Romney et al., 1985
Cervix	189 cases 227 controls	Reduced risk with increased vitamin C intake	Verreault et al., 1989
Cervix	513 cases 490 controls	No effect of dietary vitamin C	Marshall et al., 1983

[a]Severe dysplasia or carcinoma in situ

Table 3 (continued)

Site	Subjects	Findings	Reference
Pancreas	99 cases 301 controls	Reduced risk with (frequent) citrus fruit consumption	Norell et al., 1986
Prostate	311 cases 294 controls	Increased risk associated with high vitamin C intake in men over 70 years of age	Graham et al.,1983
Prostate	418 cases 771 controls	No effect of dietary vitamin C	Kolonel et al., 1985
Prostate	181 cases 181 controls	No effect of dietary vitamin C	Heshmat et al., 1985
Colon	256 cases 783 controls	Reduced risk with increased cruciferous vegetable consumption	Graham et al., 1978
Colon	102 cases 361 controls	Reduced risk with increased dietary vitamin C	Heilbrun et al., 1989
Colorectal	542 cases 1077 controls	No effect of dietary vitamin C	Jain et al., 1980
Colorectal	406 cases 812 controls	Reduction in risk with increased intake of oranges, tomatoes and green peppers	Modan et al., 1981
Colorectal	419 cases 732 controls	Reduced risk of rectal cancer associated with dietary vitamin C, most strongly in women	Potter and McMichael, 1986

Site	Cases/Controls	Finding	Reference
Colorectal	1207 cases 3531 controls	Reduced risk of colon and rectal cancers associated with high vitamin C intake	Tuyns, 1986
Colorectal	715 cases 727 controls	Reduced risk for vitamin C intakes greater than 230 mg/day	Kune et al., 1987
Colorectal	11888 older adults, 126 cases	Reduced risk (in women), with increased dietary vitamin C (but not supplemented or total C)	Wu et al., 1987
Colorectal	575 cases 778 controls	No significant relationship to citrus fruit consumption	LaVecchia et al., 1988
Colon	231 cases 391 controls	No effect of dietary vitamin C	West et al., 1989
Rectum	330 cases 628 controls	No significant relationship to cruciferous vegetable consumption	Graham et al., 1978
Lung	41 cases 870 controls	Reduced risk with vitamin C intake ≥ 70 mg/day	Kromhout et al., 1987
Lung	1253 cases 1274 controls	Reduced risk with vitamin C intake ≥ 140 mg/day	Fontham et al., 1988
Lung	49 cases 98 controls	Reduced risk with vitamin C intake ≥ 50 mg/day	Holst et al., 1988
Lung	88 cases 137 controls	Reduced risk with increased dietary vitamin C	Koo, 1988
Lung	332 cases 865 controls	Reduced risk with increased dietary vitamin C (males only)	LeMarchand et al., 1989

Table 3 (continued)

Site	Subjects	Findings	Reference
Lung	2952 cases large cohort	Reduced risk with frequent fruit consumption	Long–de & Hammond, 1985
Lung	292 cases 801 controls	No effect of dietary vitamin C	Mettlin et al., 1979
Lung	33 cases cohort of 1921	No significant effect of dietary vitamin C	Shekelle et al., 1981
Lung	72 cases cohort of 16713	No significant effect of dietary vitamin C	Kvale et al., 1983
Lung	364 cases 627 controls	No significant effect of dietary vitamin C	Hinds et al., 1984
Lung	427 cases 1094 controls	No effect of dietary vitamin C	Byers et al., 1984
Lung	115 cases 308 controls	No significant association with plasma vitamin C level (prospective)	Stahelin et al., 1987

Table 4 Intervention Trials: Vitamin C and Cancer

Subjects	Vitamin C	Findings	Reference
51 patients with hypochlorhydria	4 × 1 g/day for 4 weeks	Reduction in nitrate and N-nitroso compound formation	Reed et al., 1983
8 male duodenal ulcer patients	4 × 1 g/day for 7 days	Significantly reduced mutagenicity of gastric juice without a change in pH	O'Connor et al., 1985
36 patients with polyposis coli	3 g/day or placebo for 15–24 months	Reduction in polyp area in treated group at 9 months and trend toward a reduction in number, but differences declined toward the end of the trial	Bussey et al., 1982
238 adults from areas with high or low risk of esophageal cancer	3 × 100 mg per day	Supplement reduced urinary N–nitros-amino acids in high-risk subjects to to levels found in low-risk subjects	Lu et al., 1986
24 lung and 35 bladder cancer patients	5 g/day in 3 divided doses	Increase in serum vitamin C levels from subclinical hypovitaminosis C to the upper normal range	Greco et al., 1982
100 patients with advanced colorectal cancer	10 g/day or placebo	No effect of treatment on disease prog-ression or patient survival	Moertel et al., 1985

day. Even when adjusted for other dietary variables, vitamin C intake above this threshold level was associated with about a 40% reduction in the risk of developing colorectal cancer.

Other studies have shown an association between dietary vitamin C and reduced risk of rectal (but not colon) cancer (Potter and McMichael, 1986), colon (but not rectal) cancer in men (Heilbrun et al., 1989), and colorectal cancer in women only (Wu et al., 1987). Although dietary intake of vitamin C per se was not evaluated, a reduced risk of developing colon cancer was found to be associated with high intakes of some cruciferous vegetables (Graham et al., 1978). A study of the consumption of numerous food items in relation to colorectal cancer incidence showed a reduction in risk with frequent green vegetable intake, but found no significant reduction with high fresh fruit or citrus fruit intakes (La Vecchia et al., 1988). There was also no apparent relationship between vitamin C intake and the development of colorectal cancer in an earlier study (Jain et al., 1980). These studies may have failed to show a relationship between vitamin C and colorectal cancers because the highest dietary intakes may have fallen below the critical threshold level.

An intervention trial was conducted to investigate the effect of supplemental vitamin C on polyposis coli (rectal polyps) (Bussey et al., 1982), which have the potential to evolve into malignancies (Morson, 1974). Persons receiving 3 g/day of ascorbic acid for 15–24 months showed a trend toward a reduction in size and number of the polyps during the middle of the trial, in comparison with placebo controls, but the significance failed to be maintained throughout the study. There was no statistically significant effect of supplementation with vitamins C (4 g/day) and E (400 mg/day) in a similar population, although supplementation was (nonsignificantly) negatively associated with polyp number in 14 of 16 sigmoidoscopic evaluations (DeCosse et al., 1989). Further studies of the efficacy of ascorbic acid and other micronutrients in the treatment of polyposis coli are currently underway (Bertram et al., 1987).

8. Lung Cancer

Both no effect and a strongly protective effect of vitamin C against lung cancer have been reported. Some of the early studies showed no association between vitamin C intake and lung cancer risk (Mettlin et al., 1979, Byers et al., 1984), or produced statistically insignificant evidence suggesting a protective effect of high dietary (Shekelle et al.,1981; Kvale et al.,1983; Hinds et al., 1984), or stored plasma vitamin C (Stahelin et al., 1987). However, several recent reports suggest that foods rich in vitamin C may be protective against lung cancer. A large cohort study demonstrated that frequent fresh fruit consumption was associated with reduced lung cancer risk (Long-de and Hammond, 1985). High dietary vitamin C was found to be related to reduced risk of lung cancer in women who never smoked cigarettes (Koo, 1988) and in men (but not women) (LeMarchand et al., 1989) in case-control studies. A prospective dietary study found a protective effect against lung cancer of vitamin C intakes at or above 70 mg/day; the risk associated with intakes below 60 mg/day was nearly three times higher than the risk for consumption of 100 mg/day or more (Kromhout, 1987). In other studies, intakes at or below 50 mg/day were associated with 4 times higher risk relative to greater intakes (Holst et al., 1988), and intakes below 90 mg/day correlated with almost twice the risk associated with intakes of vitamin C over 140 mg/day (Fontham et al., 1988). It is interesting to note that cigarettes smoking is correlated with both high lung cancer incidence and poor ascorbic acid status (Hoefel, 1983).

9. Other Cancer Sites

Epidemiological studies have shown relationships between high citrus fruit consumption and significantly decreased risk of developing pancreatic cancer (Norell et al., 1986), and between the frequent ingestion of vitamin C containing foods and a decreased risk of developing cancers of the mouth (Marshall et al., 1982; Winn et al., 1984; McLaughlin et al., 1988) and larynx (Graham, 1981). Retrospective case-control studies of diet found that low vitamin C intake may contribute to an increased risk of developing severe cervical dysplasia (Wassertheil-Smoller et al., 1981; Romney et al., 1985), and invasive cervical cancer (Verreault et al., 1989). Additional studies are required before conclusions can be drawn from any of these findings.

10. Summary

At present scientific evidence in support of the efficacy of vitamin C in the treatment of advanced cancer is weak. There are numerous proposed mechanisms by which vitamin C may be useful in reducing the risk of developing certain types of cancer. The epidemiological evidence suggests that a high dietary intake of vitamin C and/or vitamin C-rich foods may reduce the risk of developing oral, esophageal, gastric, and colorectal cancers. There is limited evidence of a relationship between vitamin C intake and lung cancer.

B. Immune Functions

The functions of the immune system include tumor surveillance and the destruction of bacteria and viruses. Competent immune response is therefore a very important factor in the body's defense against infections and cancer. It has been hypothesized that vitamin C is immunostimulatory

(Anderson, 1984), primarily through enhancement of neutrophil function. This has led to interest in the potential beneficial effects of vitamin C in reducing the risk of cancer, in preventing or ameliorating colds, and in treating periodontal disease, chronic infections, and asthma. Vitamin C may also improve resistance to infection by stimulating collagen formation in the skin and epithelial lining of orifices, which maintain a physical barrier against pathogens (Bendich, 1987).

1.   In Vitro and Animal Studies

An important step in arresting bacterial infection is the engulfment and destruction of foreign particles by specific immune system cells (phagocytes). Studies in which human white blood cells have been incubated with ascorbic acid and bacteria indicate that the vitamin promotes phagocytic activity (*Nutrition Reviews,* 1978; Schmidt and Moser, 1985) and chemotaxis (Boxer et al., 1979). The stimulation of phagocytosis and lymphocyte motility appears to be dependent upon the vitamin C concentration outside the cells (Boxer et al., 1979).

Ascorbate may also prevent the initiation of mononuclear leukocyte suppressor activity (Eftychis and Anderson, 1983); suppressor activity reduces the strength of immune responses. In vitro work also suggests that vitamin C may reduce nitrogen-stimulated inflammation (Mirza and Amaral, 1983) and increase histamine catabolism (Sharma and Wilson, 1980). However, extremely high levels of ascorbic acid (well above normal concentrations) may inhibit natural killer cell activity (Huwyler et al., 1985).

In one study, vitamin C supplementation to guinea pigs resulted in a larger and more rapid antibody response to a cellular antigen than in unsupplemented animals (Prinz et al., 1980).

2.   Human Studies

One hour following an intravenous injection of ascorbate (1 g), blood from healthy adults showed significant increases in neutrophil motility and lymphocyte transformation (Anderson, 1981a). Vitamin C supplementation has been associated with enhancement of human leukocyte function (Shilotri and Bhat, 1977; Anderson et al., 1980) (Table 5).

In healthy older adults, intramuscular vitamin C injections (500 mg/ day for 1 month) improved lymphocyte proliferation in response to certain mitogens (in vitro) and enhanced the tuberculin skin hypersensitivity response (Kennes et al., 1983). There was also a trend toward increased response to skin tests in a group of elderly persons self-supplementing with high doses of vitamin C (Goodwin and Garry, 1983), but the difference from nonsupplementers was not significant.

Table 5 Effect of Vitamin C Suplementation on In Vitro and In Vivo Immune System Responses

Subjects	Vitamin C	Findings	Reference
5 healthy adults	200 mg and 2 g/day for 2 weeks each	In vivo: 2 g/day significantly *impaired* bacteriological activity; both levels stimulated HMPS activity in leukocytes	Shilotri and Bhat, 1977
5 healthy adults	1,2, and 3 g/day for 1 week each	Enhanced neutrophil motility in response to chemotactic stimulation at 2 and 3–g levels (in vitro). No change in immuno-globulins or complement	Anderson et al., 1980
16 healthy adults	10 g/day or placebo	Increased lymphocyte DNA synthesis in response to a mitogen with in vitro incubation in physiological levels of vita-min C but no difference between cells from supplemented and unsupplemented	Delafuente and Panush, 1980
6 healthy adults	1 g, I.V. single dose	Increase in vitro neutrophil motility and and lymphocyte transformation	Anderson, 1981
260 healthy adults 65–94 years	Self supplement-ing up to 7 g/ day	Nonsignificant trend for high dose takers to have increased mitogen responses in vivo (as measured by skin test) but not in vitro.	Goodwin and Garry 1983
20 healthy adults over 70 years of age	500 mg/day I.M. for 1 month (or saline pla-cebo)	Enhanced proliferative response of T lymphocytes to some mitogens in vitro and TB skin test in vivo. No change in immunoglobulin concentrations.	Kennes et al., 1983
12 adults (65+ years) with chronic illness	2 g/day or placebo for 3 weeks	No effect on mitogen-stimulated lymphocyte proliferation or in vivo skin test antigen response	Delafuente et al., 1986

A recent study found that healthy adults given a single 4–g dose of vitamin C had a significant increase in serum interleukin–1 and total white blood cell count (Sutor and Johnson, 1988). This suggests a potential mechanism for vitamin C in boosting disease resistance.

Vitamin C may also enhance antibacterial nonspecific immune system function. Chronic granulomatous disease (CGD) is a genetic disorder that compromises the immune system's ability to destroy pathogens. A 1 g/day dose of ascorbic acid for 2 years decreased infections, slightly increased in vitro neutrophil hexose monophosphate shunt (HMPS) activity, and improved neutrophil motility in a small group of CGD patients (Anderson, 1981b). However, others saw no in vivo benefit with supplemental vitamin C in a similar group of patients (Patrone et al., 1982).

A single infant with Chediak-Higashi syndrome, another genetic disorder affecting immune function, was treated with 1 g of ascorbic acid per day (Boxer et al., 1976). The supplementation was associated with a significant improvement in her previously impaired leukocyte bactericidal activity and chemotaxis; these parameters became abnormal again when the vitamin C dosage was discontinued. Interestingly, the supplement also significantly enhanced leukocyte chemotaxis in two normal controls (Boxer et al., 1976). Another patient with Chediak-Higashi syndrome had normalized neutrophil bactericidal activity and significantly fewer infections during 3 years of supplementation with vitamin C (Weening et al., 1981).

A small group of subjects with defective bacterial killing and consequent repeated infections were kept infection-free for 1 year with 1–2 g daily vitamin C supplementation (Rebora et al., 1980).

Chronically ill elderly subjects who were vitamin C-sufficient did not show in vivo or in vitro changes in immune response after 3 weeks of 2 g daily vitamin C supplementation or placebo (Delafuente et al., 1986).

C. Wound Healing

Vitamin C is known to be required for the formation of normal collagen. Bruising and impaired wound healing are prevalent in vitamin C-deficient humans and animals. In addition, supplemental vitamin C may accelerate wound healing in the absence of a clinical deficiency (Ringsdorf and Cheraskin, 1982).

Although decreases in blood ascorbic acid levels have been consistently reported in postoperative patients (with no increase in excretion of the vitamin) (Shulka, 1969; Irvin et al., 1978), there is controversy over the clinical significance of this finding. Some researchers maintain that the drop represents increased need, whereas others suggest that ascorbic acid is redistributed to tissues (Schorah et al., 1986). It has been observed that the use of general anesthesia decreases plasma ascorbic acid (Akita et al., 1987), although the reason for this is unclear. The tissue ascorbic acid concentration at the site of a wound has been found to increase (Crandon et al., 1961). Similarly, the change in blood vitamin C following surgery may be artifactual, resulting from changes in leukocyte ratios (Vallance, 1986). Nonetheless, studies have shown significant reductions in healing time and wound opening with high-dose vitamin C supplementation (Crandon et al., 1961). Some investigators have found a dose-response improvement in these healing parameters with increased vitamin C supplementation (Schwartz, 1970).

D. Cardiovascular Health

Vitamin C has been studied as a factor in cardiovascular health. Cardiovascular disease is largely associated with atherosclerosis, the formation of fatty plaques within the wall of blood vessels. Atherosclerotic plaques can be initiated when the vessel wall is damaged, such as through oxidative injury or mechanical stress. Because vitamin C is involved in collagen formation, antioxidant protection, and certain cellular reactions that facilitate fat metabolism, a possible role for ascorbate in ameliorating atherosclerosis has been hypothesized. Nonetheless, mechanisms by which vitamin C may influence cardiovascular health have yet to be established.

1. Serum Lipids

Serum cholesterol levels are highly correlated with heart disease. Low–density lipoproteins (LDL) circulate in the blood with a high proportion of cholesterol (LDL–C) and are thought to contribute to plaque formation. By contrast, high-density lipoproteins (HDL) "scavenge" cholesterol, and high levels of HDL are associated with a reduced risk of cardiovascular disease.

Much of the controversy over the possible benefit of high vitamin C intake in relation to cardiovascular health is based on studies of serum cholesterol. Studies with animals suggest that vitamin C stimulates the activity of cholesterol 7–alpha–hydroxylase (Holloway and Rivers, 1981; Holloway et al., 1984), the enzyme regulating the conversion of cholesterol to bile acids. Since bile acids are the vehicle for cholesterol excretion, vitamin C might in turn lower blood cholesterol concentrations. The reports are controversial, and vitamin C intake does not consistently correlate with total serum cholesterol in humans (Lapidus et al., 1986). The beneficial effect of vitamin C may be through an increase in HDL, the so–called "good" cholesterol, rather than through a lowering of total cholesterol (TC). It has been suggested that vitamin C significantly alters cholesterol levels only in hypercholesterolemic subjects (Ginter et al., 1977). Others have theorized that vitamin C mobilizes the cholesterol in arterial walls, thereby improving the condition of the arteries without significantly lowering (and sometimes even raising) serum lipid levels (Spittle, 1974).

A number of studies have attempted to evaluate the effect of vitamin C supplementation on serum HDL and/or total cholesterol. Many of the studies showed no positive effect of vitamin C supplementation on serum lipids. These studies, however, were mainly conducted for short periods of time (Spittle, 1971; Joshi et al.,1981; Khan and Seedarnee, 1981; Wahlberg and Walldius, 1982; Burr et al., 1985), with small study populations (Peterson et al., 1975; Johnson and Obenshain, 1981; Khan and Seedarnee, 1981; Wahlberg and Walldius, 1982), or in people with very high initial serum ascorbic acid levels (mean levels of 1.3 mg/dl or higher) (Peterson et al., 1975, Johnson and Obenshain 1981; Elliott 1982) (Table 6).

Positive correlations between serum ascorbic acid level and HDL–C have been reported in several studies in healthy men but not women (Bates et al., 1977), and in another study in both men and women over 60 years of age (Jacques et al., 1987a) (Table 7). An inverse correlation between serum ascorbic acid and total cholesterol was seen in a group of male smokers (Kevany et al., 1975). However, in other studies, no correlation was seen between vitamin C status and serum lipids in healthy older Americans (Hooper et al., 1983) or Nigerian nomads (Ette and Kale, 1986).

2. Blood Pressure

High blood pressure (hypertension) is considered a major risk factor for cardiovascular disease.

An evaluation of the first Health and Nutrition Examination Survey (NHANES I) data shows that people with lower vitamin C consumption had higher blood pressure (McCarron et al., 1984). A study of apparently healthy men in their 30s found a strong inverse association between serum ascorbic acid level and high blood pressure (Yoshioka et al., 1984) (Table 8). The same relationship was seen in a large study of 54–year–old Finnish men (Salonen et al., 1988). Plasma ascorbic acid levels were inversely associated with resting blood pressure, and mean blood pressure was substantially higher among those with low plasma vitamin C (less than 0.4 mg/dl) compared with those with the highest plasma levels of the vitamin (Salonen et al., 1988). However, no significant association was seen between vitamin C intake and systolic blood pressure in a group of Swedish women (Lapidus et al., 1986). A daily 1–g supplement of vitamin C to mildly hypertensive women was associated with drops in both systolic and diastolic blood pressure, as well as lower plasma lipids (Koh, 1984).

3. Platelets

A critical stage in the development of atherosclerosis is platelet aggregation and adhesion following injury to vessel walls. An injury stimulates the
production of prostaglandins such as thromboxane, which cause the platelet aggregation and clotting. This platelet response and the accompanying
prostaglandin production are associated with a burst of oxidation reactions. Another prostaglandin, prostacyclin, protects vessel walls from
platelet accumulation.

Studies in animals have shown that atherosclerosis induced by a high
cholesterol diet can be prevented or reversed by a high vitamin C intake
(Altman et al., 1980). Vitamin C may have its beneficial effect in these animal models through a reported increase in prostacyclin production
(Beetens and Herman, 1983; Beetens et al., 1986), reducing platelet aggregation. Ascorbic acid may also reduce platelet activity by hampering the
platelet release mechanism (Cowan et al., 1975).

In humans, an acute dose of ascorbic acid (2 g, injected intravenously)
caused an inhibition of platelet aggregation in vitro and reduced the concentration of malondialdehyde, a product of oxidation reactions, in platelets (Cordova et al., 1982). In another study individuals with existing coronary artery disease (CAD) were given either placebo, 1 g, or 2 g of vitamin
C (in two daily doses), for 6 months (Bordia, 1980). At the higher ascorbic
acid dose there was a significant increase in fibrinolytic activity (which is
thought to be a factor in clearing arteries) and a 27% decrease in an index
of platelet adhesiveness (Bordia,1980). The subjects, who were mildly hyperlipidemic, also had a significant drop in serum total cholesterol while on
the 2 g/day vitamin C supplementation. In addition, the increase in platelet aggregation and adhesiveness induced in CAD patients by a high-cho-
lesterol meal was prevented by the addition of 1 g of ascorbic acid to the
food (Bordia and Verma, 1985). The ingestion of 1 g of vitamin C every 8
hours for 10 days significantly reduced platelet aggregation and adhesion
in a group of hyperlipidemic CAD patients who had had abnormally high
measures of these parameters (Bordia and Verma, 1985). However, one
study reported no effect of 1 g/day ascorbic acid treatment on platelet adhesiveness (Crawford et al., 1975). This may indicate that a high threshold
level of ascorbic acid is required to influence platelet activity. It has been
suggested that a daily 1 g dose of vitamin C is the minimum necessary to be
protective against thrombotic disease (Spittle, 1974).

4. Stroke

Cerebrovascular strokes are associated with atherosclerosis and hypertension. Lipid peroxides have also been implicated in the etiology of
strokes (Huang et al., 1988). As discussed above, vitamin C may influence

Table 6 Summary of Studies on the Effects of Vitamin C Supplementation on Serum Lipoprotein Cholesterol and Total Cholesterol (TC)

Subjects	Vitamin C	Duration	Findings	Reference
			I. Positive Effects	
58 healthy men and women	1 g/day	6 weeks	TC tended to fall only in those subjects under 25	Spittle, 1971
25 patients with atherosclerosis	1 g/day	6 weeks	Significant upward trend in TC level with supplement	Spittle, 1971
82 men and women aged 50–75 yrs.	500mg twice a day +20mg from food	3 months	Significant decrease in TC, most change in subjects with higher initial cholesterolemia	Ginter et al., 1977
48 stabilized, hyper-cholesterolemic diabetics	500mg/day	1 year	Substantial drop in TC and moderate decline in TG, initial serum AA lower in diabetics than controls	Ginter et al., 1978
11 adults with ischemic heart disease and 14 controls	1 g/day	6 weeks	Significant rise in HDL-C in all men, reduced TC and LDL-C in men with IHD; HDL-C rose and TG decreased in women with IHD	Horsey et al., 1981
23 mildly hyperten-sive women	1 g/day	3 months	Significant decrease in TG, VLDL-C; less significant decrease in blood pressure	Koh, 1984
50 healthy adult students	2 g/day	2 months	Significant decrease in TC and and increase in HDL-C	Erden et al., 1985a
25 women aged 60–100 years and 20 controls	200mg twice a day + 60mg from food	2 years	Significant decrease in TC and an increase in HDL-C	Ziemlanski et al., 1986

II. No Significant Effects

Subjects	Dose	Duration	Effect	Reference
27 healthy men aged 17–20 years	30mg/kg/day (about 2g/day)	20 days	No significant effect on serum TC or HDL-C	Joshi et al., 1981
9 healthy men aged 20–40 years	1g/day	12 weeks	No significant effect on serum TC, HDL-C, TG or LDL-C	Johnson and Oben-shain, 1981
13 healthy women aged 21–28 years	1g/day	4 weeks	No significant effect on TC, TG, HDL-C, LDL-C or VLDL-C	Khan and Seedarnee, 1981
9 patients with hypertriglyceridemia	1g twice a day	1 month	No significant effect on TC, TG or lipoprotein fractions	Wahlberg & Walldius, 1982
9 hypercholesterolemic men & women	4g/day	2 months	No significant change in plasma cholesterol or TG	Peterson et al. 1975
26 men & women aged 25–76 years	1g three times a day	12 weeks	No significant effect on TC, HDL-C, TG or bile acids	Elliott, 1982
22 patients with arteriosclerosis obliterans	1g/day	3 months	No significant effect on TC, HDL, LDL or TG	Norden et al., 1984
50 diabetics with elevated serum lipids	500mg/day	4 months	No significant difference from placebo in TG or TC.	Bishop et al., 1985
130 healthy men aged 65–74 years	150mg/day	6 weeks	No significant effect on serum TC or HDL-C	Burr et al., 1985
24 smokers and 59 nonsmokers (young males)	0, 100 or 1000 mg/day	90 days	No consistent changes, although TC was higher in those with low AA status	Bazzarre, 1986

Table 7 Summary of Studies on an Association between Vitamin C Status/Intake and Serum Lipoprotein Cholestrol and Total Cholesterol

Subjects	Vitamin C	Duration	Findings	Reference
41 middle-aged male smokers	Blood sample and survey of smoking habits	—	Significant correlations between ascorbic acid (AA) and serum total cholestrol (TC)	Kevany et al., 1975
23 healthy men and women aged 72–86 years	Quarterly blood samples and dietary intake	18 months	Strong positive correlation between HDL-C and plasma AA in men, weaker association with dietary-AA; no correlation between AA status and TC	Bates et al., 1977
761 men and women aged 60–100 years	Two 3-day food records and plasma samples	—	Plasma AA significantly correlated with HDL-C but not TC. Strongest in youngest (60–69 years)	Jacques et al., 1987a
			No Effect	
270 healthy men and women aged 60–93 years	Blood sample and 3-day food record	—	No correlation between AA intake or plasma AA and TG, TC, HDL-C or LDL-C	Hooper et al., 1983
102 healthy Nigerian nomads	Blood sample	—	No correlation between AA status and cholestrol level	Ette and Kale, 1986

Table 8 Association between Serum Ascorbic Acid Level and Blood Pressure and Prevalence of Hypertension (140/90 mm Hg and above) in Males Aged 30–39

Serum ascorbic acid level (mg/dl) (mean)	No. of subjects (mean age ± SD)	Systolic BP (mm Hg± SD)	Diastolic BP (mm Hg ± SD)	Prevalence of hypertension (frequency relative to high C group)
≤0.5 (0.48)	51 (36.1 ± 3)	121.9 ± 10***	77.5 ± 8**	9 (7.41*)
0.6 – 0.8 (0.76)	101 (34.9 ± 2)	118.0 ± 10**	76.1 ± 9*	11 (4.57)
≥0.9 (1.06)	42 (35.3 ± 2)	113.2 ± 10	72.8 ± 7	1 (1.00)

*p < 0.05, **p < 0.01, ***p < 0.001, significant difference in comparison with high serum ascorbic acid level group.
Source: Adapted from Yoshioka et al., 1984.

Table 3 Epidemiological Studies: Vitamin C And Cancer Risk

Site	Subjects	Findings	Reference
Oral/ Pharyngeal	227 cases 405 controls	Reduced risk with more frequent fruit and vegetable intake	Winn et al., 1984
Oral/ Pharyngeal	871 cases 979 controls	Reduced risk with increased fruit intake, vitamin C intake	McLaughlin et al., 1988
Oral	425 cases 588 controls	Reduced risk (dose-response) as vitamin C intake increased	Marshall et al., 1982
Pharyngeal	166 cases 547 controls	Reduced risk with increased vitamin C intake	Rossing et al., 1989
Larynx	374 cases 381 controls	Reduced risk with increased vitamin C intake	Graham et al., 1981
Esophagus	344 cases 688 controls	Reduced risk with increased intake of fresh fruit and raw vegetables	Cook-Mozaffari et al., 1979
Esophagus	120 cases 250 controls	Reduced risk with increased intake of vitamin C-rich foods	Ziegler et al., 1981
Esophagus	147 cases 264 controls	Reduced risk (dose-response) with increased ingestion of foods containing vitamin C	Mettlin et al., 1981
Esophagus	743 cases 1975 controls	Reduced risk with increased vitamin C and citrus fruit intake	Tuyns et al., 1987
Stomach	228 cases 1394 controls	Reduced risk associated with high vitamin C intake in people < 60 years old	Bjelke, 1974
Stomach	391 cases 391 controls	Reduced risk with increased fruit and dietary vitamin C.	Correa et al., 1985

Stomach	246 cases 246 controls	Reduced risk with increased citrus fruit but total vitamin C intake less protective	Risch et al., 1985
Stomach	110 cases 100 cases	Reduced risk with increased lemon and orange consumption	Trichopoulos et al., 1985
Stomach	206 cases 474 controls	Reduced risk with increased fresh fruit, specifically citrus	LaVecchia et al., 1987
Stomach	564 cases 1131 controls	Reduced risk associated with greater dietary intake of vitamin C	You et al., 1988
Stomach	267 men from low- and 246 from high-risk towns	Plasma ascorbate and fruit intake were lower in the high-risk area but no direct relationship between ascorbate and atrophic gastritis	Burr et al., 1987
Stomach	188 cases 800 controls	No difference between cases and controls in frequency of citrus fruits/juice consumption	Graham et al., 1967
Bladder	164 cases 314 controls	Reduced risk with increased vitamin C intake in most groups	Kolonel et al., 1985
Cervix[a]	32 cases 71 controls	Reduced risk with vitamin C intake above the median (76 mg/day)	Wassertheil-Smoller et al. 1981
Cervix[a]	17 cases 34 controls	Reduced risk with increased serum ascorbate levels	Romney et al., 1985
Cervix	189 cases 227 controls	Reduced risk with increased vitamin C intake	Verreault et al., 1989
Cervix	513 cases 490 controls	No effect of dietary vitamin C	Marshall et al., 1983

[a]Severe dysplasia or carcinoma in situ

Table 3 (continued)

Site	Subjects	Findings	Reference
Pancreas	99 cases 301 controls	Reduced risk with (frequent) citrus fruit consumption	Norell et al., 1986
Prostate	311 cases 294 controls	Increased risk associated with high vitamin C intake in men over 70 years of age	Graham et al.,1983
Prostate	418 cases 771 controls	No effect of dietary vitamin C	Kolonel et al., 1985
Prostate	181 cases 181 controls	No effect of dietary vitamin C	Heshmat et al., 1985
Colon	256 cases 783 controls	Reduced risk with increased cruciferous vegetable consumption	Graham et al., 1978
Colon	102 cases 361 controls	Reduced risk with increased dietary vitamin C	Heilbrun et al., 1989
Colorectal	542 cases 1077 controls	No effect of dietary vitamin C	Jain et al., 1980
Colorectal	406 cases 812 controls	Reduction in risk with increased intake of oranges, tomatoes and green peppers	Modan et al., 1981
Colorectal	419 cases 732 controls	Reduced risk of rectal cancer associated with dietary vitamin C, most strongly in women	Potter and McMichael, 1986

Site	Cases/Controls	Finding	Reference
Colorectal	1207 cases 3531 controls	Reduced risk of colon and rectal cancers associated with high vitamin C intake	Tuyns, 1986
Colorectal	715 cases 727 controls	Reduced risk for vitamin C intakes greater than 230 mg/day	Kune et al., 1987
Colorectal	11888 older adults, 126 cases	Reduced risk (in women), with increased dietary vitamin C (but not supplemented or total C)	Wu et al., 1987
Colorectal	575 cases 778 controls	No significant relationship to citrus fruit consumption	LaVecchia et al., 1988
Colon	231 cases 391 controls	No effect of dietary vitamin C	West et al., 1989
Rectum	330 cases 628 controls	No significant relationship to cruciferous vegetable consumption	Graham et al., 1978
Lung	41 cases 870 controls	Reduced risk with vitamin C intake $\geq$ 70 mg/day	Kromhout et al., 1987
Lung	1253 cases 1274 controls	Reduced risk with vitamin C intake $\geq$ 140 mg/day	Fontham et al., 1988
Lung	49 cases 98 controls	Reduced risk with vitamin C intake $\geq$ 50 mg/day	Holst et al., 1988
Lung	88 cases 137 controls	Reduced risk with increased dietary vitamin C	Koo, 1988
Lung	332 cases 865 controls	Reduced risk with increased dietary vitamin C (males only)	LeMarchand et al., 1989

Table 3 (continued)

Site	Subjects	Findings	Reference
Lung	2952 cases large cohort	Reduced risk with frequent fruit consumption	Long–de & Hammond, 1985
Lung	292 cases 801 controls	No effect of dietary vitamin C	Mettlin et al., 1979
Lung	33 cases cohort of 1921	No significant effect of dietary vitamin C	Shekelle et al., 1981
Lung	72 cases cohort of 16713	No significant effect of dietary vitamin C	Kvale et al., 1983
Lung	364 cases 627 controls	No significant effect of dietary vitamin C	Hinds et al., 1984
Lung	427 cases 1094 controls	No effect of dietary vitamin C	Byers et al., 1984
Lung	115 cases 308 controls	No significant association with plasma vitamin C level (prospective)	Stahelin et al., 1987

Table 4 Intervention Trials: Vitamin C and Cancer

Subjects	Vitamin C	Findings	Reference
51 patients with hypochlorhydria	4×1 g/day for 4 weeks	Reduction in nitrate and N–nitroso compound formation	Reed et al., 1983
8 male duodenal ulcer patients	4×1 g/day for 7 days	Significantly reduced mutagenicity of gastric juice without a change in pH	O'Connor et al., 1985
36 patients with polyposis coli	3 g/day or placebo for 15–24 months	Reduction in polyp area in treated group at 9 months and trend toward a reduction in number, but differences declined toward the end of the trial	Bussey et al., 1982
238 adults from areas with high or low risk of esophageal cancer	3×100 mg per day	Supplement reduced urinary N–nitros-amino acids in high-risk subjects to to levels found in low-risk subjects	Lu et al., 1986
24 lung and 35 bladder cancer patients	5 g/day in 3 divided doses	Increase in serum vitamin C levels from subclinical hypovitaminosis C to the upper normal range	Greco et al., 1982
100 patients with advanced colorectal cancer	10 g/day or placebo	No effect of treatment on disease progression or patient survival	Moertel et al., 1985

Table 5 Effect of Vitamin C Suplementation on In Vitro and In Vivo Immune System Responses

Subjects	Vitamin C	Findings	Reference
5 healthy adults	200 mg and 2 g/day for 2 weeks each	In vivo: 2 g/day significantly *impaired* bacteriological activity; both levels stimulated HMPS activity in leukocytes	Shilotri and Bhat, 1977
5 healthy adults	1,2, and 3 g/day for 1 week each	Enhanced neutrophil motility in response to chemotactic stimulation at 2 and 3–g levels (in vitro). No change in immuno-globulins or complement	Anderson et al., 1980
16 healthy adults	10 g/day or placebo	Increased lymphocyte DNA synthesis in response to a mitogen with in vitro incubation in physiological levels of vita-min C but no difference between cells from supplemented and unsupplemented	Delafuente and Panush, 1980
6 healthy adults	1 g, I.V. single dose	Increase in vitro neutrophil motility and and lymphocyte transformation	Anderson, 1981
260 healthy adults 65–94 years	Self supplement-ing up to 7 g/ day	Nonsignificant trend for high dose takers to have increased mitogen responses in vivo (as measured by skin test) but not in vitro.	Goodwin and Garry 1983
20 healthy adults over 70 years of age	500 mg/day I.M. for 1 month (or saline pla-cebo)	Enhanced proliferative response of T lymphocytes to some mitogens in vitro and TB skin test in vivo. No change in immunoglobulin concentrations.	Kennes et al., 1983
12 adults (65+ years) with chronic illness	2 g/day or placebo for 3 weeks	No effect on mitogen-stimulated lymphocyte proliferation or in vivo skin test antigen response	Delafuente et al., 1986

Table 6 Summary of Studies on the Effects of Vitamin C Supplementation on Serum Lipoprotein Cholesterol and Total Cholesterol (TC)

Subjects	Vitamin C	Duration	Findings	Reference
			I. Positive Effects	
58 healthy men and women	1 g/day	6 weeks	TC tended to fall only in those subjects under 25	Spittle, 1971
25 patients with atherosclerosis	1 g/day	6 weeks	Significant upward trend in TC level with supplement	Spittle, 1971
82 men and women aged 50–75 yrs.	500mg twice a day +20mg from food	3 months	Significant decrease in TC, most change in subjects with higher initial cholesterolemia	Ginter et al., 1977
48 stabilized, hyper-cholesterolemic diabetics	500mg/day	1 year	Substantial drop in TC and moderate decline in TG; initial serum AA lower in diabetics than controls	Ginter et al., 1978
11 adults with ischemic heart disease and 14 controls	1 g/day	6 weeks	Significant rise in HDL-C in all men, reduced TC and LDL-C in men with IHD; HDL-C rose and TG decreased in women with IHD	Horsey et al., 1981
23 mildly hyperten-sive women	1 g/day	3 months	Significant decrease in TG, VLDL-C; less significant decrease in blood pressure	Koh, 1984
50 healthy adult students	2 g/day	2 months	Significant decrease in TC and and increase in HDL-C	Erden et al., 1985a
25 women aged 60–100 years and 20 controls	200mg twice a day + 60mg from food	2 years	Significant decrease in TC and an increase in HDL-C	Ziemlanski et al., 1986

Table 8 Association between Serum Ascorbic Acid Level and Blood Pressure and Prevalence of Hypertension (140/90 mm Hg and above) in Males Aged 30–39

Serum ascorbic acid level (mg/dl) (mean)	No. of subjects (mean age ± SD)	Systolic BP (mm Hg± SD)	Diastolic BP (mm Hg ± SD)	Prevalence of hypertension (frequency relative to high C group)
≤0.5 (0.48)	51 (36.1 ± 3)	121.9 ± 10***	77.5 ± 8**	9 (7.41*)
0.6 – 0.8 (0.76)	101 (34.9 ± 2)	118.0 ± 10**	76.1 ± 9*	11 (4.57)
≥0.9 (1.06)	42 (35.3 ± 2)	113.2 ± 10	72.8 ± 7	1 (1.00)

*p < 0.05, **p < 0.01, ***p < 0.001, significant difference in comparison with high serum ascorbic acid level group.
Source: Adapted from Yoshioka et al., 1984.

all of these determinants, i.e., atherosclerosis, hypertension and lipid peroxides, and may therefore be a factor in the risk of stroke. A rise in the leukocyte ascorbic acid of supplemented elderly subjects was associated with a lower number of pinpoint hemorrhages (caused by a blood pressure cuff), in comparison with subjects receiving a placebo (Eddy, 1972). It has been suggested that low vitamin C levels increase the fragility of arteries and capillaries, and when coupled with hypertension, may lead to hemorrhages and stroke (Taylor, 1976).

Acheson and Williams (1983), noting an association between a declining cerebrovascular disease (CVD) rate and an increase in fruit and vegetable consumption in Britain and the United States, have proposed that these foods may be protective against stroke. The authors suggest that the reduced risk of CVD associated with eating fresh fruit and vegetables may be due to their vitamin C content (Acheson and Williams, 1983). They also point out that fresh produce is a good source of potassium, a factor in hypertension risk (McCarron et al., 1984; Tobian, 1988), although the reduced risk of CVD mortality associated with eating fruit and vegetables was strengthened when foods were weighted for their ascorbic acid content (Vollset and Bjelke, 1983).

5. Conclusions

Numerous studies, cited above, provide evidence for an association between vitamin C and cardiovascular health. Leukocyte ascorbic acid was reported to be significantly lower in patients with coronary artery disease than in normals (Ramirez and Flowers, 1980). A 12–year follow-up study of Swedish women found a negative correlation between vitamin C intake and serum triglycerides, body mass index, and waist-to-hip circumference ratio—all cardiovascular disease risk factors (Lapidus et al., 1986). A cross-cultural epidemiological study found an association between lower vitamin C status and medium to high rates of coronary mortality (Gey et al., 1987). These findings suggest that vitamin C, possibly through its effects on HDL cholesterol, blood pressure, and/or platelets, may improve cardiovascular health and reduce the risk of cardiovascular mortality.

E. Cataracts

When proteins in the lens of the eye are oxidized, they polymerize and cause cloudiness that interferes with vision. This occurs during the formation of cataracts. Lens proteins turn over very slowly, over decades, and are exposed to large amounts ultraviolet light, which predisposes them to oxidative damage. This oxidation may be a causal factor in cataract formation (Taylor, 1989), and in fact, cataracts are more common and progress more rapidly in countries with comparatively strong sunlight exposure (Varma et al., 1984).

The human lens has a high concentration of antioxidant enzymes and ascorbic acid. The levels of these antioxidants in the lens decrease (Ohrloff et al., 1984) and the incidence of cataract increases with age. In addition, as cataracts develop, vitamin C content of the lens declines (Lohmann, 1987). Human cataractous lenses have been found to contain less than half the concentration of ascorbic acid found in normal lenses (Chandra et al., 1986). In vitro work indicates that vitamin C protects the lens by inhibiting lipid photoperoxidation (Varma et al., 1984).

In a retrospective study, Jacques et al., (1987b) reported a lower incidence of cataract in subjects whose ascorbic acid intake was in the highest quintile (probability of cataract, 0.24), compared with those in the lowest quintile (probability defined as 1.00).

Vitamin supplement use was studied in 175 people with cataracts and 175 controls (Robertson et al., 1989). Subjects who took no supplement had a relative risk of developing cataracts four times higher than did subjects self-supplementing with vitamin C (300–600 mg/day) (Robertson et al., 1989 see chapter 5, Table 7).

F. Iron Absorption

There are two types of dietary iron sources, heme iron (from the hemoglobin and myoglobin found in meats) and nonheme iron (from other sources such as plants, cooking utensils, and drinking water). Nonheme iron, which constitutes the major portion of dietary iron intake (Monsen, 1988), is very poorly absorbed. In some diets only 3% of the nonheme iron is absorbed while up to 23% of the iron present in the form of heme is absorbed (Monsen, 1988). When consumed with a meal, vitamin C markedly increases nonheme iron absorption (Kuhn et al., 1968), but has little or no effect on heme iron availability. The absorption of non–heme iron from a vegetarian meal containing 74 mg of vitamin C was estimated to be twice as high as that from a meal containing a similar amount of iron but only 14 mg of vitamin C (Hallberg and Rossander, 1982). The addition of 60 mg of ascorbic acid to a rice meal increased iron absorption from 3.2% to 11.9% (Sayers et al., 1974). On average, 25–75 mg of ascorbic acid is required to achieve significantly greater iron absorption (Monsen et al., 1978; Monsen, 1988). Hallberg (1981) estimates that the addition of 50–100 mg of ascorbic acid to meals doubles or triples nonheme iron absorption. In order to facilitate iron absorption, vitamin C needs to be consumed along with the meal (Figure 1).

Iron intake is likely to be inadequate in the U.S. population during infancy, rapid growth phases, adolescence, pregnancy, and in premenopausal women (Committee on Dietary Allowances, 1980). Iron deficiency anemia is a significant world health problem (International Nutritional Anemia Consultative Group, 1977). The prevalence of anemia in the U.S. population, based on NHANES II data, was found to be 5.7% in infants, 5.9% in teenage girls, 5.8% in young women, and 4.4% in elderly men (Dallman et al., 1984). Vitamin C supplementation to anemic young children in India significantly raised hemoglobin levels and improved other indices of anemia in the Philippines (Aguilar, 1983), India (Seshadri et al., 1985), and China (Wen-guang et al., 1986).

Since excessive iron loading is potentially toxic, the effects of vitamin C supplementation on iron stores have been investigated. Interestingly, vitamin C deficiency and low vitamin C status have been associated with

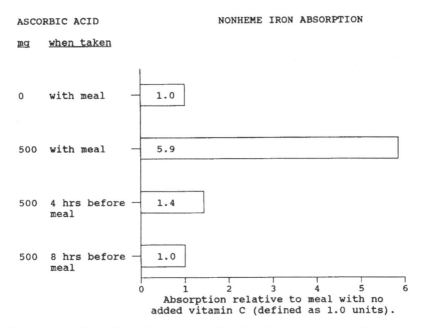

Figure 1   The effect of ascorbic acid administration on nonheme iron absorption. *Source*: Adapted from Monsen, E. R., Fig. 3, *J. Am. Diet. Assoc.* *88*:786 (1988); based on data from Cook and Monsen (1977).

iron overload (Roeser, 1983; *Nutrition Reviews,* 1987). This is apparently due to accelerated breakdown of ascorbic acid in the presence of high iron concentrations, and to the role of the vitamin in mobilizing iron stores (Roeser, 1983). In fact, while simultaneous vitamin C and iron ingestion increases the percent of iron absorbed from the gut in normal subjects, high-dose vitamin C therapy is associated with lower serum ferritin (a measure of iron status) in certain cases of iron overload (Tagliabue et al., 1984). Although 2 g/day vitamin C supplementation with meals increased the absorption of nonheme iron by fivefold in a group of healthy adults (Cook et al., 1984), the supplement did not alter long-term iron stores. Similarly, 125 mg/day ascorbic acid supplementation (not taken with meals) did not alter serum ferritin concentration in normal men and women (Tagliabue et al., 1985) (the vitamin C must be present in the gut *at the same time* as the iron in order to increase its absorption). It was concluded that the body's mechanism of iron balance adapts appropriately to varied iron intake and absorption (Cook et al., 1984; Tagliabue et al., 1985).

G. Bone Metabolism

Severe bone loss (osteoporosis) appears to be the result of a constellation of nutritional, genetic, and physiological factors and is most commonly seen in small-sized, older Caucasian females.

One of the nutrients involved in bone metabolism is ascorbic acid. Vitamin C is required for the synthesis of strong collagen, which forms the structural framework of bone. Cases of infant scurvy are associated with epiphyseal separation and abnormalities in cartilage formation leading to impaired bone formation; in fact, infantile scurvy was historically confused with rickets (Clemetson, 1989). In addition, in vitro work suggests that ascorbic acid may have a direct influence on bone cell growth, independently of its effect on collagen formation (Sugimoto et al., 1986).

In one study, osteoporosis (indicated by vertebrae collapse) in apparently healthy Bantu men was found to be associated with iron overload (which causes accelerated vitamin C destruction) and low leukocyte ascorbic acid levels (Lynch et al., 1967). Men in this population consumed large quantities of iron and very little fresh fruit and had a high incidence of scurvy and osteoporosis. A postmortem study on a comparable group revealed an association between low ascorbic acid status and low bone density (Lynch et al., 1967).

Both bone density and vitamin C status decline with increasing age (Moriuchi and Hosoya, 1985). Estrogen seems to be protective against bone loss, and as a result, postmenopausal women are at particular risk for developing osteoporosis. Several studies have shown a correlation between ascorbic acid intake and bone mineral content or bone density in postmenopausal women (Freudenheim et al., 1986; Sowers et al., 1985) and in a mixed population (Odland et al., 1972).

These findings are consistent with those of animal studies. Scorbutic guinea pigs have been found to have increased bone loss, similar to that seen in osteoporosis, with impaired bone matrix formation and cessation of bone growth (Poal-Manresa et al., 1970). When osteoporosis is experimentally induced in guinea pigs, supplemental vitamin C reduces the severity of damage to joints (Schwartz et al., 1981).

A human trial found that high-dose vitamin C administration (5 g twice a day for 5 days) did not significantly alter 24–hour urinary calcium excretion, although there was a significant increase in excretion within 8 hours of taking a single 2–g dose (Tsao et al., 1986).

These findings suggest that in humans intake of even large doses (5 g) of vitamin C does not adversely affect calcium balance. A study showing adverse effects of high vitamin C intake on calcium balance in guinea pigs may have used an unreasonably excessive dose (equivalent to 350 mg/day in a human), coupled with poor magnesium intake (Bray and Briggs, 1984). Ascorbic acid intake at moderate dose levels is important and safe for bone maintenance, and therefore a factor in mitigating or delaying osteoporosis.

H. Periodontal Disease

Periodontal diseases are associated with, and exacerbated by opportunistic infectious agents which are endemic in the U. S. population. In the United States, approximately 85% of adults have some periodontal disease (U.S. Department of Health and Human Services, 1986). The most common periodontal disease is periodontitis, which begins with inflammation of the gums (gingivitis) and which leads to bone resorption and tooth loss, if left unchecked.

1. Causes and Contributing Factors in Periodontal Disease

Periodontal disease is a multifactorial condition. However, poor oral hygiene and reduced host resistance are considered the major etiological factors. Pathogenic bacteria in dental plaque, and the toxins they produce, infiltrate and damage the susceptible periodontium. Impairment of tissue replacement and repair, reduced salivary gland functions, poor diet, and tobacco use are additional factors that contribute to periodontal disease.

2. Vitamin C and Periodontal Health

Because bleeding gums and loosened teeth are classical symptoms of scurvy, vitamin C status has historically been associated with periodontal health. This has led to investigations into the relationship between vitamin C and gum disease. Many early studies in this area, however, were poorly controlled and inconclusive (Ismail et al., 1983). More recent controlled studies do suggest a critical role for vitamin C in periodontal health at intakes much higher than the usual recommendations (Aurer–Kozelji et al., 1982; Buzina et al., 1986; Leggott et al., 1986).

Analysis of the first National Health and Nutrition Examination Survey data indicated a weak but significant relationship between low dietary intake of vitamin C and a high index of periodontal disease in people who reported that they did not take nutritional supplements (Ismail et al., 1983). However, differences in income levels and oral hygiene status obscure the association. Also, it is not possible to distinguish cause and effect, since peridontal disease may alter appetite and eating ability.

In another recent study, gum biopsies from individuals with low plasma ascorbic acid levels (0.18–0.30 mg/dl) were found to have damaged connective tissue. However, following the use of a 70-mg daily supplement of vitamin C, electron microscopy revealed increased collagen bundles and intracellular linkages (Aurer–Kozelj et al., 1982). Vitamin C supplementation significantly increased hydroxyproline and proline concentrations (an indicator of collagen content) in periodontal tissue; a plasma vitamin C level of 0.9 mg/dl appeared to be the threshold level (Buzina et al., 1986). The optimal plasma level was found to be 1.00–1.30 mg/dl.

Vitamin C depletion in humans under well–controlled conditions was associated with significantly increased probed gum bleeding, even though no clinical symptoms of scurvy were seen in any subject (Leggott et al., 1986). A decrease in bleeding was seen with ascorbic acid repletion: supplements of 600 mg/day were associated with a greater improvement than supplemental intakes of 60 mg/day. The degree of gingival inflammation was directly related to ascorbic acid status (Leggott et al., 1986).

3.   Scientific Rationale for a Role of Vitamin C in Periodontal Disease

Several lines of evidence suggest that vitamin C may reduce the risk of periodontal disease. Vitamin C is required for the formation of collagen, which is critical in maintaining tissue integrity and resistance to microbial invasion. Ascorbic acid appears to play a role in maintaining the cementing structures between buccal epithelial cells in guinea pigs (Thaete and Grim, 1974). Bacterial infiltration of periodontal tissues can be resisted by an optimal immune response, particularly neutrophil chemotaxis and bactericidal activity. Sufficient levels of vitamin C could therefore also reduce the risk of periodontal disease because the vitamin has been shown to enhance leukocyte chemotaxis (Boxer et al., 1979; Anderson, 1981a) and other immune system functions (Anderson, 1984) (see Section B). Further, it has been hypothesized that poor vitamin C status may aggravate gingivitis through excessive histamine production, leading to continual inflammation (Nakamoto et al., 1984). Thus there is a strong scientific rationale for a protective effect of vitamin C against periodontal disease.

4. Risk Groups

A number of groups are at risk for periodontal disease and also for inadequate vitamin C status, such as the elderly, diabetics (Schneir et al., 1985), smokers (Rivera-Hidalgo, 1986), and oral contraceptive users (Pearlman, 1974).

I. Colds

The efficacy of high dose vitamin C supplementation in preventing or ameliorating the so-called "common cold" has been controversial (Preshaw, 1972; Jaffe, 1984). Numerous studies have been conducted in this area (Table 9). Reviewers have variously concluded that, on balance, these studies show no significant health benefit associated with ascorbic acid supplementation (Schwartz et al., 1973; Dykes and Meier, 1975; Coulehan, 1979), or that the data indicate a beneficial effect on colds, primarily in reducing their severity (Pauling, 1971; Anderson et al., 1972; Wilson and Loh, 1973; *Nutrition Reviews,* 1973; Anderson, 1979).

Protocols for nearly all of the studies of vitamin C and colds are open to significant criticisms. In the majority of cases, subjects were free-living and exposed to a wide variety of infectious organisms of varying virulence, and many were self-reporting both symptoms and compliance. Other confounding factors in the study designs included small sample sizes, poor control of total vitamin C intake by all subjects, use of multivitamins with ascorbic acid as placebos, and administration of the vitamin only after onset of a cold. One of the most significant problems with these studies is the failure to determine the vitamin C status of the subjects initially or during treatment.

A number of variables were controlled in one study in which still no benefit of vitamin C supplementation was seen (Schwartz et al., 1973). However, in this study the viral inoculation used to cause infection was overwhelming and might have negated the benefit, if any, of vitamin C. In addition, supplementation was associated with only moderate increases in serum ascorbic acid levels, due either to poor compliance or to individual physiological variability.

Recently, a well-controlled, double-blind placebo trial of vitamin C prophylaxis and colds was conducted (Mink et al., 1988). Subjects were isolated and exposed to a single type of rhinovirus (rhinovirus type 16) through contact with an infected person. The group receiving vitamin C

(500 mg four times a day) experienced half the degree of symptom severity seen in the placebo group. Vitamin-supplemented subjects had significant increases in serum ascorbic acid levels, whereas those receiving placebo had a substantial decline in vitamin C status. This study supports the hypothesis that there is a beneficial role for vitamin C in the treatment and/or prevention of the common cold. Additional trials are necessary to clarify the role of vitamin C in this controversial area.

III. SAFETY

It has been claimed that ingestion of vitamin C in excessive quantities can contribute to kidney stone formation (Sestili, 1983), conditioning and rebound scurvy (Basu, 1985), vitamin B_{12} destruction (Herbert and Jacob, 1974), mutagenicity (Stich et al., 1976), impaired copper utilization (Finley and Cerklewski, 1983), abnormal psychological function (Benton, 1981), iron overload (McLaran et al., 1982) (see Iron Aborption), transient diarrhea, and laboratory testing errors. Only the latter two effects appear to be supported by some published literature (Hornig and Moser, 1981; Rivers, 1987).

High intakes of ascorbic acid were postulated to contribute to kidney stone formation because oxalate, a component of stones, is produced during catabolism of the vitamin and because vitamin C may acidify urine. However, oxalate formation appears to be a saturable system (Schmidt et al., 1981), and in hyperoxalurics, oxalate that is produced from vitamin C is insignificant in comparison with oxalate from dietary sources (Atkins et al., 1965; Hagler and Herman, 1973). In addition, numerous studies have shown no indication that high doses of vitamin C do, in fact, increase the incidence of kidney stone formation (Schmidt et al., 1981; Sutton et al., 1983; Hoffer, 1985; Erden et al., 1985b; Singh et al., 1988). It may nonetheless be prudent for individuals with renal insufficiency or who have a tendency to form kidney stones to limit sources of oxalate, including vitamin C.

Incidences of "rebound scurvy," the appearance of scorbutic symptoms following the withdrawal of high-dose vitamin C intake, have been largely anecdotal. There has been no experimental evidence for such an effect in humans (Hornig and Moser, 1981; Gerster and Moser, 1988). Guinea pig studies in this area have been negative or inconclusive (Rivers, 1987).

The finding that large amounts of ascorbic acid destroyed vitamin B_{12} was shown to be an artifact of the experimental method (Marcus et al., 1980). The assertion that vitamin C is mutagenic also resulted from an error in in vitro methodology (Norkus et al., 1983).

TABLE 9 Summary of Studies on Vitamin C and the Common Cold Intervention Studies: 1942–1988

Reference	Double blind	Randomized	Placebo-controlled	Baseline serum C	Final serum C	Same viral infection	Direct inoculum	Dietary C estimated	Compliance measured	Number of subjects	Daily C intake (g)	C on sick days (g)	Treatment duration (days)	Reduced incidence	Reduced duration	Reduced severity	Comments
Cowan et al., 1942	•	•	•					•	•	427	0.1 & 0.2	0.5	196	•			Urine tested for C
Dahlberg et al., 1944	•	•	•	a	a					2525	0.05		90				
Cowan & Diehl, 1950	•	•	•							367		0.667	180				
Macon, 1956		•	a						•	121		0.05	4			•	All got aspirin
Tebrock et al., 1956	•	•	a							1900	0.2[a]	0.2	3				All got aspirin
Barnes, 1961		•	•							39	3	3	49				Part of multivitamin
Walker et al., 1967	•	•	•			•				91			9	•	•		
GP Research Group, 1968	•	•	•							270	3	3	14				
Anderson et al., 1972	•	•	•							818	1	4	60–90	a	a		Not significant
Schwartz et al., 1973	•	•	•	•	•	•	•			21	3		28				All were made ill

Study	Subjects	Dose			Comments
Wilson et al., 1973	302	0.2		270	
Anderson et al., 1974	2349	1	4	90	Other tx combinations
Coulehan et al., 1974	641	1 & 2		90–150	
Anderson et al., 1975	448	0.5/wk	1	105	Only incidence rated
Carson et al., 1975	244	1		80	
Clegg and Macdonald, 1975	211	1		105	d-isoascorbate, not C
Karlowski et al., 1975	190	3	6	270	Subjects broke blind
Coulehan et al., 1976	856	1		105–24	
Elwood et al, 1976	688	1		100	Only chest colds↓
Elwood et al, 1977	1082		3	3	Benefit in men only
Ludvigsson et al., 1977	615	0.01/1		90	
Miller et al., 1977	88	0.5–1		150	Cotwin study
Tyrrell et al., 1977	1501		4	2 1/2	
Baird et al., 1979	350	0.08		72	
Pitt et al., 1979	674	2		54	
Carr et al., 1981	190	1		100	
Cartolano et al., 1981	686	0.5		90	Cotwin study
Briggs, 1984	516	0.05/1	0.2/4	90–120	
Mink et al., 1988	16	2		45	

C = vitamin C; • = yes; ↓ = reduced; ª See note in comments column.

Controlled studies have shown no support for claims that high ascorbic acid intake impairs psychological performance (Pascoe and Stone, 1984) or copper absorption (Jacob et al., 1987b; Milne et al., 1988).

IV. SUMMARY

Epidemiological evidence suggests that vitamin C-rich foods may reduce the risk of developing cancers of the gastrointestinal tract.

In vitro and animal studies indicate that vitamin C may have a role in enhancing immune function. Ascorbic acid supplementation has been associated with improvement in certain indices of immune response in human subjects.

Adequate vitamin C status is necessary for the formation of collagen, a critical step in wound healing and bone and blood vessel formation.

Supplemental vitamin C may reduce risk factors for cardiovascular disease by increasing levels of high-density lipoproteins, and by reducing total cholesterol in hyperlipidemic individuals. There is additional, albeit limited, evidence that a high intake of vitamin C may be efficacious in reducing blood pressure, inhibiting platelet aggregation, and lowering risk of stroke.

A high vitamin C status has been associated with a reduced risk of cataract development, possibly through a reduction in the oxidative destruction of lens proteins.

When both nutrients are present simultaneously in the gut, vitamin C improves nonheme iron absorption.

There is evidence that adequate intake of vitamin C would reduce the risk of periodontal disease. Some recent findings suggest that the need for vitamin C as judged by periodontal health may be more than the current RDA— about 100 mg/day.

Earlier evidence of the efficacy of vitamin C in treatment or prevention of the common cold was equivocal. However, many of the studies had serious design flaws. The preliminary report of a recent, carefully controlled investigation suggests that vitamin C may reduce the severity of cold symptoms.

Because adverse effects of oral vitamin C supplementation have not been convincingly demonstrated, even at intakes as high as 10–20 g/day, a safe upper limit cannot be defined.

REFERENCES

Acheson, R. M. and Williams, D. R. R. (1983). Does consumption of fruit and vegetables protect against stroke? *Lancet 1*:1191–1193.

Aguilar, J. R. (1983). Asorbic acid supplementation and vitamin A fortification of anemic Filipino children and its effect on iron nutriture. Diss. Cornell University.

Akita, S., Kawahara, M., Takeshita, T., Morio, M. and Fujii, K. (1987). Effect of general anesthesia on plasma ascorbic acid level. *Hiroshima J. Med. Sci. 36*: 69–73.

Altman, R. F. A., Schaeffer, G. M. V., Salles, C. A., Ramos de Souza, A. S., and Cotias, P. M. T. (1980). Phospholipids associated with vitamin C in experimental atherosclerosis. *Drug Res. 30*:627–630.

Anderson, R. (1981a). Ascorbate-mediated stimulation of neutrophil motility and lymphocyte transformation by inhibition of the peroxidase/H_2O_2/halide system in vitro and in vivo. *Am. J. Clin. Nutr. 34*:1906–1911.

Anderson, R. (1981b). Assessment of oral ascorbate in three children with chronic granulomatous disease and defective neutrophil motility over a 2-year period. *Clin. Exp. Immunol. 43*:180–188.

Anderson, R. (1984). The immunostimulatory, anti-imflammatory and anti-allergic properties of ascorbate. In *Advances in Nutritional Research*, vol. 6, H. H. Draper (Ed). Plenum Press, New York, pp. 19– 45.

Anderson, R., Oosthuizen, R., Maritz, R., Theron, A., and Van Rensburg, A. J. (1980). The effects of increasing weekly doses of ascorbate on certain cellular and humoral immune functions in normal volunteers. *Am. J. Clin. Nutr. 33*:71–76.

Anderson, T. W. (1979). Vitamin C: cure for the common cold? *Am. Pharmacy 19*:46– 48.

Anderson, T. W., Reid, D. B. W., and Beaton, G. H. (1972). Vitamin C and the common cold: a double-blind trial. *Can. Med. Assoc. J. 107*: 503–508.

Anderson, T. W., Suranyi, G., and Beaton, G. H. (1974). The effect on winter illness of large doses of vitamin C. *Can. Med. Assoc. J. 111*(1):31–6.

Anderson, T. W., Beaton, G. H., Corey, P., and Spero, L. (1975). Winter illness and vitamin C: the effect of relatively low doses. *Can Med. Assoc. J. 112*(7):823–6.

Atkins, G. L., Dean, B. M., Griffin, W. J., Scowen, E. F., and Watts, R. W. E. (1965). Quantitative aspects of ascorbic acid metabolism in patients with primary hyperoxaluria. *Clin. Sci. 29*:305–314.

Aurer-Kozelj, J., Kralj-Klobucar, N., Buzina, R., and Bacic, M. (1982). The effect of ascorbic acid supplementation on periodontal tissue ultrastructure in subjects with progressive periodontitis. *Int. J. Vit. Nutr. Res. 52*:333–341.

Baird, I. M., Hughes, R. E., Wilson, H. K., et al. (1979). The effects of ascorbic acid and flavonoids on the occurrence of symptoms normally associated with the common cold. *Am. J. Clin. Nutr. 32*(8):1686–1690.

Barnes, F. E. (1961). Vitamin supplements and incidence of colds in high school basketball players. *NC Med. J. 22*:22.

Basu, T. K. (1985). The conditioning effect of large doses of ascorbic acid in guinea pigs. *Can. J. Physiol. Pharmacol. 63*:427– 430.

Basu, T. K. and Schorah, C. J. (1982). *Vitamin C in Health and Disease.* AVI Publishing Co. Westport, CT, pp. 61–92.

Bates, C. J., Mandal, A. R., and Cole, T. J. (1977). H. D. L. cholesterol and vitamin-C status. *Lancet 2*:611.

Bazzarre, T. L. (1986). Effects of vitamin C supplementation among male smokers and non-smokers. *Nutr. Rep. Int. 33*:711–720.

Beetens, J. R. and Herman, A. G. (1983). Vitamin C increases the formation of prostacyclin by aortic rings from various species and neutralizes the inhibitory effect of 15-hydroperoxy-arachidonic acid. *Br. J. Pharmacol. 80*:249–254.

Beetens, J. R., Coene, M. C., Verheyen, A., Zonnekeyn, L., and Herman, A. G. (1986). Vitamin C increases the prostacyclin production and decreases the vascular lesions in experimental atherosclerosis in rabbits. *Prostaglandins 32*:335–352.

Bellander, T., Osterdahl, B. G., and Hagmar, L. (1988). Excretion on N-mononitrosopiperazine after low level exposure to piperazine in air: effects of dietary nitrate and ascorbate. *Toxicol. Appl. Pharmacol. 93*:281–287.

Bendich, A. (1987). Vitamin C and immune responses. *Food Technol. 41*:112–114.

Bendich, A., Machlin, L. J., Scandurra, O., Burton, G. W., and Wayner, D. D. M. (1986). The antioxidant role of vitamin C. *Adv. Free Rad. Biol. Med. 2*:419– 444.

Benton, D. (1981). The influence of large doses of vitamin C on psychological functioning. *Psychopharmacology 75*:98–99.

Bertram, J. S., Kolonel, L. N., and Meyskens, F. L., Jr. (1987). Rationale and strategies for chemoprevention of cancer in humans. *Cancer Res. 47*:3012–3031.

Bishop, N., Schorah, C. J., and Wales, J. K. (1985). The effect of vitamin C supplementation on diabetic hyperlipidaemia: a double blind, cross-over study. *Diabetic Med. 2*:121–124.

Bjelke, E. (1974). Epidemiologic studies of cancer of the stomach, colon and rectum with special emphasis on the role of diet. *Scand. J. Gastroenterol. 9*(suppl):1–235.

Block, G. and Menkes, M. (1989). Ascorbic acid in cancer prevention. In *Nutrition and Cancer Prevention: Investigating the Role of Micronutrients*, T. E. Moon and M. S. Micozzi (Eds). Marcel Dekker, New York, pp. 341–388.

Bonjour, J. P. (1979). Vitamins and alcoholism. I. Ascorbic acid. *Int. J. Vit. Nutr. Res. 49*:434– 441.

Bordia, A. K. (1980). The effect of vitamin C on blood lipids, fibrinolytic activity and platelet adhesiveness in patients with coronary artery disease. *Atherosclerosis 35*:181–187.

Bordia, A. and Verma, S. K. (1985). Effects of vitamin-C on platelet adhesiveness and platelet aggregation in coronary artery disease patients. *Clin. Cardiol. 8*:552–554.

Boxer, L. A., Watanabe, A. M., Rister, M., Besch, H. R., Allen, J., and Baehner, R. L. (1976). Correction of leukocyte function in Chediak-Higashi syndrome by ascorbate. *N. Engl. J. Med. 295*:1041–1045.

Boxer, L. A., Vanderbilt, R., Bonsib, S., Jersild, R., Yang, H. H., and Baehner, R. L., (1979). Enhancement of chemotactic response and microtubule assembly in human leukocytes by ascorbic acid. *J. Cell Physiol. 100*:119–126.

Bray, D. L. and Briggs, G. M. (1984). Decrease in bone density in young male guinea pigs fed high levels of ascorbic acid. *J. Nutr. 114*:920–928.

Briggs, M. (1984). Clinical investigation: an 8-year, prospective double-blind study of high- vs. low-dose AA supplementation for the prevention of common colds. In *Recent Vitamin Research*, M. H. Briggs (Ed). CRC Press, Boca Raton, FL, pp. 57–81.

Bryszewska, M. and Kostrzewa, E. (1987). Ascorbic acid content in plasma and erythrocytes of insulin-dependent diabetic patients. *Med. Sci. Res. 15*:1277–1278.

Buiatti, E., Palli, D., DeCarli, A., Amadori, D., Avellini, C., Bianchi, S., Biserni, R., Cipriani, F., Cocco, P., Giacosa, A., Marubini, E., Puntoni, R., Vindigni, C., Fraumeni, J., and Blot, W. (1989). A case-control study of gastric cancer and diet in Italy. *Int. J. Cancer 44*:611–616.

Burr, M. L., Bates, C. J., Goldberg, G., and Butland, B. K. (1985). Vitamin C and cholesterol in the elderly. *Hum. Nutr. Clin. Nutr. 39C*:387–388.

Bussey, H. J. R., DeCosse, J. J., Deschner, E. E., Eyers, A. A., Lesser, M. L., Morson, B. C., Ritchie, S. M., Thomson, J. P. S., and Wadsworth, J. (1982). A randomized trial of ascorbic acid in polyposis coli. *Cancer 50*:1434–1439.

Buzina, R., Aurer-Kozelj, J., Srdak-Jorgic, K., Buhler, E., and Gey, K. F. (1986). Increase of gingival hydroxyproline and proline by improvement of ascorbic acid status in man. *Int. J. Vit. Nutr. Res. 56*:367–372.

Byers, T., Vena, J., Mettlin, C., Swanson, M., and Graham, S. (1984). Dietary vitamin A and lung cancer risk: an analysis by histologic subtypes. *Am. J. Epidemiol. 120*:769–776.

Calabrese, E. J. (1985). Does exposure to environmental pollutants increase the need for vitamin C? *J. Environment Pathol. Toxicol. Oncol. 5*:81–90.

Cameron, E. and Pauling, L. (1978). Supplemental ascorbate in the supportive treatment of cancer: reevaluation of prolongation of survival times in terminal human cancer. *Proc. Natl. Acad. Sci. USA 75*:4538– 4542.

Cartolano, V., Adler, I., Autullo, G., DelIntento, M., and Salazar, D. (1981). El acido ascorbico de accion sostenida en bajas dosis reduce la incidencia de afecciones respiratorias en el invierno. *Press Med. Argent. 68*:461– 468.

Carr, A. B., Einstein, R., Lai, L. Y., Martin, N. G., and Starmer, G. A. (1981). Vitamin C and the common cold: a second MZ cotwin control study. *Acta Gent. Med. Gemellol. 30*:249–55.

Carson, M., Cox, H., Corbett, M., and Pollitt, N. (1975). Vitamin C and the common cold. *J. Soc. Occup. Med. 25*:99–102.

Chandra, D. B., Varma, R., Ahmad, S., and Varma, S. D. (1986). Vitamin C in the human aqueous humor and cataracts. *Int. J. Vit. Nutr. Res. 56*:165–168.

Chen, M. S. Hutchinson, M. L., Pecoraro, R. E., Lee, W. Y. L., and Labbe, R. F. (1983). Hyperglycemia-induced intracellular depletion of ascorbic acid in human mononuclear leukocytes. *Diabetes 32*:1078–1081.

Clegg, K. M. and Macdonald, J. M. (1975). L-Ascorbic acid and D-isoascorbic acid in a common cold survey. *Am. J. Clin. Nutr. 28*(9):973–6.

Clemetson, C. A. B. (1989). *Vitamin C*, vol. II. CRC Press, Boca Raton, FL, p. 71.

Committee on Dietary Allowances, Food and Nutrition Board (1980). *Recommended Dietary Allowances*, 9th rev. ed. National Academy of Sciences, Washington, DC.

Connelly, T. J., Becker, A., and McDonald, J. W. (1982). Bachelor scurvy. *Int. J. Dermatol. 21*:209–211.

Cook, J. D. and Monsen, E. R. (1977). Vitamin C, the common cold, and iron absorption. *Am. J. Clin. Nutr. 30*(2):235– 41.

Cook, J. D., Watson, S. S., Simpson, K. M., Lipschitz, D. A., and Skikne, B. S. (1984). The effect of high ascorbic acid supplementation on body iron stores. *Blood 64*:721–726.

Cook-Mozaffari, P. J., Azordegan, F., Day, N. E., Ressicaud, A., Sabai, C., and Aramesh, B. (1979). Oesophageal cancer studies in the Caspian

Littoral of Iran: results of a case-control study. *Br. J. Cancer 39*: 293–309.

Cordova, C., Musca, A., Viola, F., Perrone, A., and Alessandri, C. (1982). Influence of ascorbic acid on platelet aggregation in vitro and in vivo. *Atherosclerosis 41*:15–19.

Correa, P. (1985). Mechanisms of gastric carcinogenesis. In *Diet and Human Carcinogenesis*, J. V. Joossens et al. (Eds). Elsevier, New York, pp. 109–115.

Correa, P., Haenszel, W., Cuello, C., Tannenbaum, S., and Archer, M. (1975). A model for gastric cancer epidemiology. *Lancet 2*:58–60.

Correa, P., Fontham, E., Pickle, L. W., Chen, V., Lin, Y., and Haenszel, W. (1985). Dietary determinants of gastric cancer in south Louisiana inhabitants. *J. Natl. Cancer Inst. 75*:645–654.

Coulehan, J. L. (1979). Ascorbic acid and the common cold: reviewing the evidence. *Postgrad. Med. 66*:153–160.

Coulehan, J. L., Reisinger, K. S., Rogers, K. D., and Bradley, D. W. (1974). Vitamin C prophylaxis in a boarding school. *N. Engl. J. Med. 290*:6–10.

Coulehan, J. L., Eberhard, S., Kapner, L., Taylor, F., Rogers, K., and Garry, P. (1976). Vitamin C and acute illness in Navajo school children. *N. Engl. J. Med. 295*: 973–977.

Cowan, D. W. and Diehl, H. S. (1950). Antihistaminic agents and ascorbic acid in the early treatment of the common cold. *J. Am. Med. Assoc. 143*:421–424.

Cowan, D. W., Diehl, H. S., and Baker, A. B. (1942). Vitamins for the prevention of colds. *J. Am. Med. Assoc. 120*:1268–71.

Cowan, D. W., Graham, R. C., Jr., Shook, P., and Griffin, R. (1975). The influence of ascorbic acid on platelet structure and function. *Thrombos. Diathes. Haemorrh. 34*:50–62.

Crandon, J. H., Lennihan, R., Jr., Mikal, S., and Reif, A. E. (1961). Ascorbic acid economy in surgical patients. *Ann. NY Acad. Sci. 92*:246–267.

Crawford, G. P. M., Warlow, C. P., Bennett, B., Dawson, A. A., Douglas, A. S., Kerridge, D. F., and Ogston, D. (1975). The effect of vitamin C supplements on serum cholesterol, coagulation, fibrinolysis and platelet adhesiveness. *Atherosclerosis 21*:451–454.

Dahlberg, G., Engel, A., and Rydin, H. (1944). Value of ascorbic acid as a prophylactic against "common colds." *Acta Med. Scand. 119*:540–61.

Dallman, P. R., Yip, R., and Johnson, C. (1984). Prevalence and causes of anemia in the United States, 1976 to 1980. *Am. J. Clin. Nutr. 39*:437–445.

Dawson, E. B., Harris, W. A., and Powell, L. C. (1988). Apparent differences in nutritional status due to work environment. *FASEB J. 2*: A1431.

DeCosse, J. J., Miller, H. H., and Lesser, M. L. (1989). Effect of wheat fiber and vitamins C and E on rectal polyps in patients with familial ademomatous polyposis. *J. Natl. Cancer Inst.* *81*:1290–1297.

Delafuente, J. C., Prendergast, J. M., and Modigh, A. (1986). Immunologic modulation by vitamin C in the elderly. *Int. J. Immunopharmacol.* *8*:205–211.

Dykes, M. H. M. and Meier, P. (1975). Ascorbic acid and the common cold: evaluation of its efficacy and toxicity. *J. Am. Med. Assoc.* *231*:1073–1079.

Eddy, T. P. (1972). A study of the relationship between Hess tests and leucocyte ascorbic acid in a clinical trial. *Br. J. Nutr.* *27*:537–542.

Eftychis, H. and Anderson, R. (1983). Prevention of induction of suppressor activity in human mononuclear leukocytes by ascorbate and cysteine in vitro. *Int. J. Vit. Nutr. Res.* *53*:398–401.

Elliott, H. C. (1982). Effects of vitamin C loading on serum constituents in man. *Proc. Soc. Exp. Biol. Med.* *169*:363–367.

Elwood, P. C., Lee, H. P., St. Leger, A. S., Baird, M., and Howard, A. N. (1976). A randomized controlled trial of vitamin C in the prevention and amelioration of the common cold. *Br. J. Prev. Soc. Med.* *30*:193–6.

Ellwood, P. C., Hughes, S. J., and Leger, A. S. (1977). A randomized controlled trial of the therapeutic effect of vitamin C in the common cold. *Practitioner* *218*:133–137.

Erden, F., Gulenc, S., Torun M., Kocer, Z., Simsek, B., and Nebioglu, S. (1985a). Ascorbic acid effect on some lipid fractions in human beings. *Acta Vitaminol. Enzymol.* *7*:131–138.

Erden, F., Hacisalihoglu, A., Kocer, Z., Simsek, B., and Nebioglu, S. (1985b). Effects of vitamin C intake on whole blood plasma, leucocyte and urine ascorbic acid and urine oxalic acid levels. *Acta Vitaminol. Enzymol.* *7*:123–130.

Ette, S. I. and Kale, O. O. (1986). Studies on ascorbic acid and cholesterol levels in Nigerian nomadic groups. *Trop. Geogr. Med.* *38*:6–10.

Faizallah, R., Morris, A. I., Krasner, N., and Walker, R. J. (1986). Alcohol enhances vitamin C excretion in the urine. *Alcohol Alcoholism* *21*:81–84.

Fazio, V., Flint, D. M., and Wahlqvist, M. L. (1981). Acute effects of alcohol on plasma ascorbic acid in healthy subjects. *Am. J. Clin. Nutr.* *34*:2394–2396.

Finley, E. B. and Cerklewski, F. L. (1983). Influence of ascorbic acid supplementation on copper status in young adult men. *Am. J. Clin. Nutr.* *37*:553–556.

Fontham, E., Zavala, D., Correa, P., Rodriguez, E., Hunter, F., Haenszel, W., and Tannenbaum, S. R. (1986). Diet and chronic atrophic gastritis: a case-control study. *J. Natl. Cancer Inst.* 76:621–627.

Fontham, E. T. H., Pickle, L. W., Haenszel, W., Correa, P., Lin, Y., and Falk, R. T. (1988). Dietary vitamins A and C and lung cancer risk in Louisiana. *Cancer* 62:2267–2273.

Frei, B., England, L., and Ames, B. N. (1989). Ascorbate is an outstanding antioxidant in human blood plasma. *Proc. Natl. Acad. Sci. USA* 86:6377–6381.

Freudenheim, J. L., Johnson, N. E., and Smith, E. L. (1986). Relationships between usual nutrient intake and bone-mineral content of women 35-65 years of age: longitudinal and cross-sectional analysis. *Am. J. Clin. Nutr.* 44:863–876.

Garland, W. A., Kuenzig, W., Rubio, F., Kornychuk, H., Norkus, E. P., and Conney, A. H. (1986). Urinary excretion of nitrosodimethylamine and nitrosoproline in humans: interindividual and intraindividual differences and the effect of administered ascorbic acid and alpha-tocopherol. *Cancer Res.* 46:5392–5400.

Garry, P. J., Goodwin, J. S., Hunt, W. C., and Gilbert, B. A. (1982). Nutritional status in a healthy elderly population: vitamin C. *Am. J. Clin. Nutr.* 36:332–339.

Geesin, J. C., Darr, D., Kaufman, R., Murad, S., and Pinnell, S. R. (1988). Ascorbic acid specifically increases type I and type III procollagen messanger RNA levels in human skin fibroblasts. *J. Invest. Dermatol.* 90:420– 424.

General Practitioner Research Group (1968). Ineffectiveness of vitamin C in treating coryza. *Practitioner* 200:442–5.

Gerster, H. and Moser, U. (1988). Is high-dose vitamin C intake associated with systemic conditioning? *Nutr. Res.* 8:1327–1332.

Gey, K. F., Brubacher, G. B., and Stahelin, H. B. (1987). Plasma levels of antioxidant vitamins in relation to ischemic heart disease and cancer. *Am. J. Clin. Nutr.* 45:1368–1377.

Ghosh, J. and Das, S. (1985). Evaluation of vitamin A and C status in normal and malignant conditions and their possibile role in cancer prevention. *Jpn. J. Cancer Res. (Gann)* 76:1174–1178.

Ginter, E. and Chovathova, V. (1983). Vitamin C and diabetes mellitus. *Nutr. Health* 2:3–11.

Ginter, E, Cerna, O., Budlovsky, J., Balaz, V., Hruba, F., Roch, V., and Sasko, E. (1977). Effect of ascorbic acid on plasma cholesterol in humans in a long-term experiment. *Int. J. Vit. Nutr. Res.* 47:123–134.

Ginter, E., Zdichynec, B., Holzerova, O., Ticha, E., Kobza, R., Koziakova, M., Cerna, O., Ozdin, L., Hruba, F., Novakova, V., Sasko, E., and

Gaher, M. (1978). Hypocholesterolemic effect of ascorbic acid in maturity-onset diabetes mellitus. *Int. J. Vit. Nutr. Res.* *48*:368–373.

Glatthaar, B. E., Hornig, D. H., and Moser, U. (1986). The role of ascorbic acid in carcinogenesis. *Adv. Exp. Med. Biol.* *206*:357–377.

Goodwin, J. S. and Garry, P. J. (1983). Relationship between megadose vitamin supplementation and immunological function in a healthy elderly population. *Clin. Exp. Immunol.* *51*:647–653.

Graham, S. (1983). Results of case-control studies of diet and cancer in Buffalo, New York. *Cancer Res.* *43*:2409s–2413s.

Graham, S., Lilienfeld, A. M., and Tidings, J. E. (1967). Dietary and purgation factors in the epidemiology of gastric cancer. *Cancer* *20*:2224–2234.

Graham, S., Dayal, H., Swanson, M., Mittelman, A., and Wilkinson, G. (1978). Diet in the epidemiology of cancer of the colon and rectum. *J. Natl. Cancer Inst.* *61*:709–714.

Graham, S., Mettlin, C., Marshall, J., Priore, R., Rzepka, T., and Shedd, D. (1981). Dietary factors in the epidemiology of cancer of the larynx. *Am. J. Epidemiol.* *113*:675–680.

Greco, A. M., Gentile, M., Di Filippo, O., and Coppola, A. (1982). Study of blood vitamin C in lung and bladder cancer patients before and after treatment with ascorbic acid: a preliminary report. *Acta Vitaminol. Enzymol.* *4*:155–162.

Hagler, L. and Herman, R. H. (1973). Oxalate metabolism. II. *Am. J. Clin. Nutr.* *26*:882–889.

Hallberg, L. (1981). Effect of vitamin C on the bioavailability of iron from food, In *Vitamin C (Ascorbic Acid)*, J. N. Counsell, and D. H. Hornig, (Eds). Applied Science Publishers, Englewood, NJ, pp. 49–61.

Hallberg, L. and Rossander, L. (1982). Absorption of iron from Western-type lunch and dinner meals. *Am. J. Clin. Nutr.* *35*:502–509.

Halliwell, B., Wasil, M., and Grootveld, M. (1987). Biologically significant scavenging of the myeloperoxidase-derived oxidant hypochlorous acid by ascorbic acid. *Fed. Eur. Biochem. Soc.* *213*:15–18.

Heilbrun, L. K., Nomura, A., Hankin, J. H., and Stemmermann, G. N. (1989). Diet and colorectal cancer with special reference to fiber intake. *Int. J. Cancer* *44*:1–6.

Herbert, V. and Jacob, E. (1974). Destruction of vitamin B_{12} by ascorbic acid. *J. Am. Med. Assoc.* *230*:241–242.

Heshmat, M. Y., Kaul, L., Kovi, J., et al. (1985). Nutrition and prostate cancer: a case-control study. *Prostate* *6*:7–17.

Hinds, M. W., Kolonel, L. N., Hankin, J. H., and Lee, J. (1984). Dietary vitamin A, carotene, vitamin C and risk of lung cancer in Hawaii. *Am. J. Epidemiol.* *119*:227–237.

Hoefel, O. S. (1983). Smoking: an important factor in vitamin C deficiency. *Int. J. Vit. Nutr. Res.* 24:121–124.

Hoffer, A. (1985). Ascorbic acid and kidney stones. *Can. Med. Assoc. J.* 132:320.

Hoffmann, D. and Brunnemann, K. D. (1983). Endogenous formation of N-nitrosoproline in cigarette smokers. *Cancer Res.* 43:5570–5574.

Holloway, D. E. and Rivers, J. M. (1981). Influence of chronic ascorbic acid deficiency and excessive ascorbic acid intake on bile acid metabolism and bile composition in the guinea pig. *J. Nutr.* 111:412– 424.

Holloway, D. E., Guiry, V. C., Holloway, B. A., and Rivers, J. M. (1984). Influence of dietary ascorbic acid on cholesterol 7-alpha-hydroxylase activity in the rat. *Int. J. Vit. Nutr. Res.* 54:333–337.

Holst, P. A., Kromhout, D., and Brand, R. (1988). For debate: pet birds as an independent risk factor for lung cancer. *Br. Med. J.* 297: 1319–1321.

Hooper, P. L., Hooper, E. M., Hunt, W. C., Garry, P. J., and Goodwin, J. S. (1983). Vitamins, lipids and lipoproteins in a healthy elderly population. *Int. J. Vit. Nutr. Res.* 53:412– 419.

Hormozdiari, H., Day, N. E., Aramesh, B., and Mahboubi, E. (1975). Dietary factors and esophageal cancer in the Caspian Littoral of Iran. *Cancer Res.* 35:3493–3498.

Hornig, D. H. and Moser, U. (1981). The safety of high vitamin C intake in man. In *Vitamin C Ascorbic Acid*, J. N. Counsell and D. H. Hornig (Eds). Applied Science Publishers, Englewood, NJ, pp. 225–248.

Horsey, J., Livesley, B., and Dickerson, J. W. T. (1981). Ischaemic heart disease and aged patients: effects of ascorbic acid on lipoproteins. *J. Hum. Nutr.* 35:53–58.

Huang, Z-S., Lu, F-J., and Lee, T-K. (1988). Correlation between serum lipid peroxides and the lesion size in cerebrovascular disease. *Clin. Chim. Acta* 173:325–330.

Huwyler, T., Hirt, A., and Morell, A. (1985). Effect of ascorbic acid on human natural killer cells. *Immunol. Lett.* 10:173–176.

International Nutritional Anemia Consultative Group (1977). *Guidelines for the Eradication of Iron Deficiency Anemia*, S. Baker, et al., (Eds). Nutrition Foundation, Washington, DC.

Irvin, T. T., Chattopadhyay, D. K., and Smythe, A. (1978). Ascorbic acid requirements in postoperative patients. *Surg. Gynecol. Obstet.* 147: 49–55.

Ismail, A. I., Burt, B. A., and Eklund, S. A. (1983). Relation between ascorbic acid intake and periodontal disease in the United States. *J. Am. Dent. Assoc.* 107:927–931.

Jacob, R. A., Skala, J. H., and Omaye, S. T. (1987a). Biochemical indices of human vitamin C status. *Am. J. Clin. Nutr. 46*:818–826.

Jacob, R. A., Skala, J. H., Omaye, S. T., and Turnlund, J. R. (1987b). Effect of varying ascorbic acid intakes on copper absorption and ceruloplasmin levels of young men. *J. Nutr. 117*:2109–2115.

Jacques, P. F., Hartz, S. C., McGandy, R. B., Jacob, R. A., and Russell, R. M. (1987a). Ascorbic acid, HDL, and total plasma cholesterol in the elderly. *J. Am. Coll. Nutr. 6*:169–174.

Jacques, P. F., Phillips, J., Chylack, L. T., McGandy, R. B., and Hartz, S. H. (1987b). Vitamin intake and senile cataract. *J. Am. Coll. Mutr. 6*:435.

Jaffe, G. M. (1984). Vitamin C. In *Handbook of Vitamins: Nutritional, Biochemical, and Clinical Aspects*, L. J. Machlin (Ed). Marcel Dekker, New York, pp. 199–244.

Jain, M., Cook, G. M., Davis, F. G., Grace, M. G., Howe, G. R., and Miller, A. B. (1980). A case-control study of diet and colo-rectal cancer. *Int. J. Cancer 26*:757–768.

Johnson, G. E. and Obenshain, S. S. (1981). Nonresponsiveness of serum high-density lipoprotein-cholesterol to high dose ascorbic acid administration in normal men. *Am. J. Clin. Nutr. 34*:2088–2091.

Joint Iran–International Agency for Research on Cancer Study Group (1977). Esophageal cancer studies in the Caspian Littoral of Iran: results of population studies—a prodrome. *J. Natl. Cancer Inst. 59*: 1127–1138.

Joshi, V. D., Joshi, L. N., and Gokhale, L. V. (1981). Effect of ascorbic acid on total and high density lipoprotein cholesterol of plasma in normal human subjects. *Indian J. Physiol. Pharmacol. 25*:348–350.

Kallner, A., Hartmann, D., and Hornig, D. (1979). Steady-state turnover and body pool of ascorbic acid in man. *Am. J. Clin. Nutr. 32*:530–539.

Kallner, A. B., Hartmann, D., and Hornig, D. H. (1981). On the requirements of ascorbic acid in man: steady-state turnover and body pool in smokers. *Am. J. Clin. Nutr. 34*:1347–1355.

Karlowski, T. R., Chalmers, T. C., Frenkel, L. D., Kapikian, A. Z., Lewis, T. L., and Lynch, J. M. (1975). Ascorbic acid for the common cold, A prophylactic and therapeutic trial. *J. Am. Med. Assoc. 231*:1038–42.

Kassouny, M. E., Coen, C. H., and Bebok, S. T. (1985). Influence of vitamin C and magnesium on calcium, magnesium and copper contents of guinea pig tissues. *Int. J. Vit. Nutr. Res. 55*:295–300.

Keith, R. E. and Mossholder, S. B. (1986). Ascorbic acid status of smoking and nonsmoking adolescent females. *Int. J. Vit. Nutr. Res. 56*: 363–366.

Kennes, B., Dumont, I., Brohee, D., Hubert, C., and Neve, P. (1983). Effect of vitamin C supplements on cell-mediated immunity in old people. *Gerontology 29*:305–310.

Kevany, J., Jessop, W., and Goldsmith, A. (1975). The effect of smoking on ascorbic acid and serum cholesterol in adult males. *Irish J. Med. Sci. 144*:474–477.

Khan, A. R. and Seedarnee, F. A. (1981). Effect of ascorbic acid on plasma lipids and lipoproteins in healthy young women. *Atherosclerosis 39*:89–95.

Koh, E. T. (1984). Effect of vitamin C on blood parameters of hypertensive subjects. *J. Okla. State Med. Assoc. 77*:177–182.

Kolonel, L. N., Hinds, M. W., Nomura, A. M. Y., Hankin, J. H., and Lee, J. (1985). Relationship of dietary vitamin A and ascorbic acid intake to the risk for cancers of the lung, bladder, and prostate in Hawaii. *Natl. Cancer Inst. Monogr. 69*:137–142.

Kromhout, D. (1987). Essential micronutrients in relation to carcinogenesis. *Am. J. Clin. Nutr. 45*:1361–1367.

Kuhn, I. N., Layrisse, M., Roche, M., Martinez, C., and Walker, R. B. (1968). Observations on the mechanism of iron absorption. *Am. J. Clin. Nutr. 21*:1184–1188.

Kune, S., Kune, G. A., and Watson, L. F. (1987). Case-control study of dietary etiological factors: the Melbourne colorectal cancer study. *Nutr. Cancer 9*:21–42.

Lapidus, L., Andersson, H., Bengtsson, C., and Bosaeus, I. (1986). Dietary habits in relation to incidence of cardiovascular disease and death in women: a 12-year follow-up of participants in the population study of women in Gothenburg, Sweden. *Am. J. Clin. Nutr. 44*:444–448.

La Vecchia, C., Negri, E., Decarli, A., D'Avanzo, B., and Franceschi, S. (1987). A case-control study of diet and gastric cancer in Northern Italy. *Int. J. Cancer 40*:484–489.

La Vecchia, C., Negri, E., Decarli, A., D'Avanzo, B., Gallotti, L., Gentile, A., and Franceschi, S. (1988). A case-control study of diet and colo-rectal cancer in Northern Italy. *Int. J. Cancer 41*:492–498.

Leaf, C. D., Vecchio, A. J., Roe, D. A., and Hotchkiss, J. H. (1987). Influence of ascorbic acid dose on *N*-nitrosoproline formation in humans. *Carcinogenesis 8*:791–795.

Leggott, P. J., Robertson, P. B., Rothman, D. L., Murray, P. A., and Jacob, R. A. (1986). The effect of controlled ascorbic acid depletion and supplementation on peridontal health. *J. Periodontol. 57*:480–485.

Lohmann, W. (1987). Ascorbic acid and cataract. *Ann. NY Acad. Sci. 498*:307–311.

Lu, S-H., Ohshima, H., Fu, H-M., Tian, Y., Li, F-M., Blettner, M., Wahren-dorf, J., and Bartsch, H. (1986). Urinary excretion of N-nitrosamino acids and nitrate by inhabitants of high-and low-risk areas for esophageal cancer in northern China: endogenous formation of nitrosoproline and its inhibition by vitamin C. *Cancer Res. 46*:1485–1491.

Ludvigsson, J., Hansson, L. O., and Tibbling, G. (1977). Vitamin C as a preventive medicine against common colds in children. *Scand. J. Infect. Dis. 9*:91–8.

Lynch, S. R., Berelowitz, I., Seftel, H. C., Miller, G. B., Krawitz, P., Charlton, R. W., and Bothwell, T. H. (1967). Osteoporosis in Johannesburg Bantu males. *Am. J. Clin. Nutr. 20*:799–807.

Macon, W. L. (1956). Citrus bioflavinoids in the treatment of the common cold. *Industr. Med. Surg. 25*:525–27.

Majumdar, S. K., Patel, S., Shaw, G. K., Aps, E. J., O'Gorman, P., and Thomson, A. D. (1983). Blood vitamin C in patients with alcoholic liver disease. *Int. J. Vit. Nutr. Res. 53*:218–219.

Mann, G. V. (1974). Hypothesis: the role of vitamin C in diabetic angiopathy. *Perspect. Biol. Med. 17*:210–217.

Marcus, M., Prabhudesai, M., and Wassef, S. (1980). Stability of vitamin B_{12} in the presence of ascorbic acid in food and serum: restoration by cyanide of apparent loss. *Am. J. Clin. Nutr. 33*:137–143.

Marshall, J., Graham, S., Mettlin, C., Shedd, D., and Swanson, M. (1982). Diet in the epidemiology of oral cancer. *Nutr. Cancer 3*:145–149.

Marshall, J. R., Graham, S., Byers, T., Swanson, M., and Brasure, J. (1983). Diet and smoking in the epidemiology of cancer of the cervix. *J. Natl. Cancer Inst. 70*:847–851.

McCarron, D. A., Morris, C. D., Henry, H. J., and Stanton, J. L. (1984). Blood pressure and nutrient intake in the United States. *Science 224*:1392–1398.

McLaran, C. J., Bett, J. H. N., Nye, J. A., and Halliday, J. W. (1982). Congestive cardiomyopathy and haemochromatosis—rapid progression possibly accelerated by excessive ingestion of ascorbic acid. *Aust. NZ J. Med. 12*:187–188.

McLaughlin, J. K., Gridley, G., Block, G., Winn, D. M., Preston-Martin, S., Schoenberg, J. B., Greenberg, R. S., Stemhagen, A., Austin, D. F., Ershow, A. G., Blot, W. J., and Fraumeni, J. F., Jr. (1988). Dietary factors in oral and pharyngeal cancer. *J. Natl. Cancer Inst. 80*:1237–1243.

McLennan, S., Yue, D. K., Fisher, E., Capogreco, C., Heffernan, S., Ross, G. R., and Turtle, J. R. (1988). Deficiency of ascorbic acid in experimental diabetes: relationship with collagen and polyol pathway abnormalities. *Diabetes 37*:359–361.

Melethil, S., Mason, W. D., and Chang, C-J. (1986). Dose-dependent absorption and excretion of vitamin C in humans. *Int. J. Pharmaceut.* *31*:83–89.

Mettlin, C., Graham, S., Priore, R., Marshall, J., and Swanson, M. (1981). Diet and cancer of the esophagus. *Nutr. Cancer 2*:143–147.

Miller, J. Z., Nance, W. E., Norton, J. A., Wolen, R. L., Griffith, R. S., and Rose, R. J. (1977). Therapeutic effect of vitamin C. A co-twin control study. *J. Am. Med. Assoc. 237*:248– 51.

Milne, D. B., Klevay, L. M., and Hunt, J. R. (1988). Effects of ascorbic acid supplements and a diet marginal in copper on indices of copper nutriture in women. *Nutr. Res. 8*:865–873.

Mink, K. A., Dick, E. C., Jennings, L. C., and Inhorn, S. L. (1988). Amelioration of rhinovirus colds by vitamin C (ascorbic acid) supplementation. In *Medical Virology VII: Proceedings of the 1987 International Symposium on Medical Virology*, L. M. DeLaMaza and E. M. Peterson (Eds). Elsevier, New York, p. 356.

Mirza, J. and Amaral, L. (1983). The effect of ascorbic acid on the human lymphocyte. *Int. J. Tissue React. 5*:141–143.

Modan, B., Cuckle, H., and Lubin, F. (1981). A note on the role of dietary retinol and carotene in human gastro-intestinal cancer. *Int. J. Cancer 28*:421– 424.

Moertel, C. G., Fleming, T. R., Creagan, E. T., Rubin, J., O'Connell, M. J., and Ames, M. M. (1985). High-dose vitamin C versus placebo in the treatment of patients with advanced cancer who have had no prior chemotherapy. *N. Engl. J. Med 312*:137–141.

Monsen, E. R. (1988). Iron nutrition and absorption: dietary factors which impact iron bioavailability. *J. Am. Diet. Assoc. 88*:786–790.

Monsen, E. R., Hallberg, L., Layrisse, M., Hegsted, D. M., Cook, J. D., Mertz, W., and Finch, C. A. (1978). Estimation of available dietary iron. *Am. J. Clin. Nutr. 31*:134–141.

Moriuchi, S. and Hosoya, N. (1985). Changes of vitamin status and calcium metabolism in aging. *J. Nutr. Sci. Vitaminol. 31*:S11– S14.

Morson, B. (1984). The polyp-cancer sequence in the large bowel. *Proc. R. Soc. Med. 67*:451– 457.

Nakamoto, T., McCroskey, M., and Mallek, H. M. (1984). The role of ascorbic acid deficiency in human gingivitis—a new hypothesis. *J. Theor. Biol. 108*:163–171.

Newberne, P. M. and Suphakarn, V. (1984). Influence of the antioxidants vitamins C and E and of selenium on cancer. In *Vitamins, Nutrition, and Cancer*, K. N. Prasad, (Ed). Krager, Basel, pp 46–67.

Newton, H. M. V., Schorah, C. J., Habibzadeh, N., Morgan, D. B., and Hullin, R. P. (1985). The cause and correction of low blood vitamin C concentrations in the elderly. *Am. J. Clin. Nutr. 42*:656–659.

Niki, E., Saito, T., and Kamiya, Y. (1983). The role of vitamin C as an antioxidant. *Chem. Lett. 1983*:631–632.

Norden, C., Heine, H., Stepanauskas, M., Schossler, W., and Singer, P. (1984). The interaction blood to vessel wall in patients with arteriosclerosis obliterans during vitamin C treatment. *Int. J. Microbiol. 3*:425.

Norell, S. E., Ahlbom, A., Erwald, R., Jacobson, G., Lindberg-Navier, I., Olin, R., Tornberg, B., and Wiechel, K-L. (1986). Diet and pancreatic cancer: a case-control study. *Am. J. Epidemiol. 124*:894–902.

Norkus, E. P. and Kuenzig, W. A. (1985). Studies on the antimutagenic activity of ascorbic acid in vitro and in vivo. *Carcinogenesis 6*:1593–1598.

Norkus, E. P., Kuenzig, W. A. , and Conney, A. H. (1983). Studies on the mutagenic activity of ascorbic acid in vitro and in vivo. *Mutation Res. 117*:183–191.

Nutrition Reviews (1973). Vitamin C and the common cold. *Nutr. Rev. 31*:303–305.

Nutrition Reviews (1978). Vitamin C and phagocyte function. *Nutr. Rev. 36*:183–185.

Nutrition Reviews (1987). Vitamin C stabilizes ferritin: new insights into iron-ascorbate interactions. *Nutr. Rev. 45*:217–218.

O'Connor, H. J., Habibzedah, N., Schorah, C. J., Axon, A. T. R., Riley, S. E., and Garner, R. C. (1985). Effect of increased intake of vitamin C on the mutagenic activity of gastric juice and intragastric concentrations of ascorbic acid. *Carcinogenesis 6*:1675–1676.

Odland, L. M., Mason, R. L., and Alexeff, A. I. (1972). Bone density and dietary findings of 409 Tennessee subjects. I. Bone density considerations. *Am. J. Clin. Nutr. 25*:905–907.

Ohrloff, C., Hockwin, O., Olson, R., and Dickinson, S. (1984). Glutathione peroxidase, glutathione reductase and superoxide dismutase in the aging. *Curr. Eye Res. 3*:109–115.

O'Keane, M., Russell, R. I., and Goldberg, A. (1972). Ascorbic acid status of alcoholics. *J. Alcohol 7*:6–11.

Pascoe, P. A. and Stone, B. M. (1984). Ascorbic acid and performance in man. *Psychopharmacology 83*:376–377.

Patrone, F., Dallegri, F., Bonvini, E., Minervini, F., and Sacchetti, C. (1982). Effects of ascorbic acid on neutrophil function, studies on normal and chronic granulomatous disease neutrophils. *Acta Vitaminol. Enzymol. 4*:163–168.

Pauling, L. (1971). Ascorbic acid and the common cold. *Am. J. Clin. Nutr.* 24:1294–1299.

Pearlman, B. A. (1974). An oral contraceptive drug and gingival enlargement: the relationship between local and systemic factors. *J. Clin. Periodontol.* 1:47–51.

Pecoraro, R. E. and Chen, M. S. (1987). Ascorbic acid metabolism in diabetes mellitus. *Ann. NY Acad. Sci.* 498:248–258.

Pelletier, O. (1977). Vitamin C and tobacco. *Int. J. Vit. Nutr. Res.* 16: 147–169.

Peterson, V. E., Crapo, P. A., Weininger, J., Ginsberg, H., and Olefsky, J. (1975). Quantification of plasma cholesterol and triglyceride levels in hypercholesterolemic subjects receiving ascorbic acid supplements. *Am. J. Clin. Nutr.* 28:584–587.

Piatkowski, J., Wiechert, P., and Ernst, K. (1986). Ascorbic acid in chronic alcoholics. *Int. J. Vit. Nutr. Res.* 56:421.

Pitt, H. A. and Costrini, A. M. (1979). Vitamin C prophylaxis in marine recruits. *J. Am. Med. Assoc.* 241:908–11.

Poal-Manresa, J., Little, K., and Trueta, J. (1970). Some observations on the effects of vitamin C deficiency on bone. *Br. J. Exp. Pathol.* 51: 372–378.

Potter, J. D. and McMichael, A. J. (1986). Diet and cancer of the colon and rectum: a case-control study. *J. Natl. Cancer Inst.* 76:557–569.

Poulter, J. M., White, W. F., and Dickerson, J. W. T. (1984). Ascorbic acid supplementation and five year survival rates in women with early breast cancer. *Acta Vitaminol. Enzymol.* 6:175–182.

Preshaw, R. M. (1972). Vitamin C and the common cold. *Can. Med. Assoc. J.* 107:479– 480.

Prinz, W., Bloch, J., Gilich, G., and Mitchell, G. (1980). A systematic study of the effect of vitamin C supplementation on the humoral immune response in ascorbate-dependent mammals. *Int. J. Vit. Nutr. Res.* 50:294–300.

Ramirez, J. and Flowers, N. C. (1980). Leukocyte ascorbic acid and its relationship to coronary artery disease in man. *Am. J. Clin. Nutr.* 33:2079–2087.

Rebora, A., Dallegri, F., and Patrone, F. (1980). Neutrophil dysfunction and repeated infections: influence of levamisole and ascorbic acid. *Br. J. Dermatol.* 102:49–56.

Reed, P. I., Summers, K., Smith, P. L. R., Walters, C. L., Bartholomew, B. A., Hill, M. J., Vennitt, S., Hornig, D., and Bonjour, J-P. (1983). Effect of ascorbic acid treatment on gastric juice nitrite and N-nitroso compound concentrations in achlorhydric subjects. *Gut* 24:492– 493.

Ringsdorf, W. M., Jr. and Cheraskin, E. (1982). Vitamin C and human wound healing. *Oral Surg.* 53:231–236.

Risch, H. A., Jain, M., Choi, N. W., Fodor, J. G., Pfeiffer, C. J., Howe, G. R., Harrison, L. W., Craib, K. J. P., and Miller, A. B. (1985). Dietary factors and the incidence of cancer of the stomach. *Am. J. Epidemiol.* 122:947–959.

Rivera-Hidalgo, R. F. (1986). Smoking and peridontal disease: a review of the literature. *J. Periodontol.* 57:617–624.

Rivers, J. M. (1987). Safety of high-level vitamin C ingestion. *Ann. NY Acad. Sci.* 498:445– 454.

Robertson, J. M., Donner, A. P., and Trevithick, J. R. (1989). Vitamin E intake and risk of cataract in humans. *Ann. NY Acad. Sci.* 570:372–382.

Roeser, H. P. (1983). The role of ascorbic acid in the turnover of storage iron. *Semin. Hematol.* 20:91–100.

Romney, S. L., Duttagupta, C., Basu, J., Palan, P. R., Karp, S., Slagle, N. S., Dwyer, A., Wassertheil-Smoller, S., and Wylie-Rosett, J. (1985). Plasma vitamin C and uterine cervical dysplasia. *Am. J. Obstet. Gynecol.* 151:976–980.

Rossing, M. A., Vaughan, T. L., McKnight, B. (1989). Diet and pharyngeal cancer. *Int. J. Cancer* 44:593–597.

Rossner, P., Cerna, M., Pokorna, D., Hajek, V., and Petr, J. (1988). Effect of ascorbic acid prophylaxis on the frequency of chromosome aberrations, urine mutagenicity and nucleolus tests in workers occupationally exposed to cytostatic drugs. *Mutation Res.* 208:149–153.

Solonen, J. T., Solonen, R., Ihanainen, M., Parviainen, M., Seppanen, R., Kantola, M., Seppanen, K., and Rauramaa, R. (1988). Blood pressure, dietary fats, and antioxidants. *Am. J. Clin. Nutr.* 48:1226–1232.

Sasaki, R., Kurokawa, T., and Tero-Kubota, S. (1983). Ascorbate radical and ascorbic acid level in human serum and age. *J. Gerontol.* 38:26–30.

Sayers, M. H., Lynch, S. R., Charlton, R. W., Bothwell, T. H., Walker, R. B., and Mayet, F. (1974). Iron absorption from rice meals cooked with fortified salt containing ferrous sulphate and ascorbic acid. *Br. J. Nutr.* 31:367–375.

Schectman, G., Byrd, J. C., and Gruchow, H. W. (1989). The influence of smoking on vitamin C status in adults. *Am. J. Public Health* 79:158–162.

Schmidt, K. and Moser, U. (1985). Vitamin C—a modulator of host defense mechanism. *Int. J. Vit. Nutr. Res.* 27(supp):363–379.

Schmidt, K-H., Hagmaier, V., Hornig, D. H., Vuilleumier, J-P., and Rutishauser, G. (1981). Urinary oxalate excretion after large intakes of ascorbic acid in man. *Am. J. Clin. Nutr.* 34:305–311.

Schneir, M., Ramamurthy, N., and Golub, L. (1985). Dietary ascorbic acid normalizes diabetes-induced underhydroxylation of nascent type I collagen molecules. *Collagen Rel. Res.* 5:415– 422.

Schorah, C. J. (1978). Inappropriate vitamin C reserves: their frequency and significance in an urban population. In *The Importance of Vitamins to Health*, T. G. Taylor (Ed). MTP Press, Lancaster, England, pp. 61–72.

Schorah, C. J., Scott, D. L., Newill, A., and Morgan, D. B. (1979). Clinical effects of vitamin C in elderly inpatients with low blood-vitamin-C levels. *Lancet* 1:403– 405.

Schorah, C. J., Habibzadeh, N., Hancock, M., and King, R. F. G. J. (1986). Changes in plasma and buffy layer vitamin C concentrations following major surgery: what do they reflect? *Ann. Clin. Biochem.* 23:566–570.

Schorah, C. J., Bishop, N., Wales, J. K., Hansbro, P. M., and Habibzadeh, N. (1988). Blood vitamin C concentrations in patients with diabetes mellitus. *Int. J. Vit. Nutr. Res.* 58:312–318.

Schvartsman, S. (1983). Vitamin C in the treatment of paediatric intoxications. *Int. J. Vit. Nutr. Res.* 24:125–129.

Schwartz, A. R., Togo, Y., Hornick, R. B., Tominaga, S., and Gleckman, R. A. (1973). Evaluation of the efficacy of ascorbic acid in prophylaxis of induced rhinovirus 44 infection in man. *J. Infect. Dis.* 128:500–505.

Schwartz, E. R., Leveille, C., and Oh, W. H. (1981). Experimentally-induced osteoarthritis in guinea pigs: effect of surgical procedure and dietary intake of vitamin C. *Lab. Animal Sci.* 31:683–687.

Schwartz, P. L. (1970). Ascorbic acid in wound healing—a review. *J. Am. Diet. Assoc.* 56:497–503.

Sergeev, A. V. (1984). [Correction of biochemical and immunologic parameters in large bowel cancer by optimal doses of retinyl acetate and ascorbic acid.] [Rus]. *B. Exp. Biol. Med.* 96:90– 92.

Seshadri, S., Shah, A., and Bhade, S. (1985). Haematologic response of anaemic preschool children to ascorbic acid supplementation. *Hum. Nutr. Appl. Nutr.* 39A:151–154.

Sestili, M. A. (1983). Possible adverse health effects of vitamin C and ascorbic acid. *Semin. Oncol.* 10:299–304.

Sharma, S. C. and Wilson, C. W. M. (1980). The cellular interaction of ascorbic acid with histamine, cyclic nucleotides and prostaglandins in the immediate hypersensitivity reaction. *Int. J. Vit. Nutr. Res.* 50:163–170.

Shilotri, P. G. and Bhat, K. S. (1977). Effect of mega doses of vitamin C on bactericidal activity of leukocytes. *Am. J. Clin. Nutr.* 30:1077–1081.

Shukla, S. P. (1969). Plasma and urinary ascorbic acid levels in the post operative period. *Experientia* 25:704.

Singh, P. P., Sharma, D. C., Rathore, V., and Surana, S. S. (1988). An investigation into the role of ascorbic acid in renal calculogenesis in albino rats. *J. Urol. 139*:156–157.

Smith, J. L. and Hodges, R. E. (1987). Serum levels of vitamin C in relation to dietary and supplemental intake of vitamin C in smokers and non-smokers. *Ann. NY Acad. Sci. 498*:144–152.

Som, S., Raha, C., and Chatterjee, I. B. (1983). Ascorbic acid: a scavenger of superoxide radical. *Acta Vitaminol. Enzymol. 5*:243–250.

Sowers, M. R., Wallace, R. B., and Lemke, J. H. (1985). Correlates of mid-radius bone density among postmenopausal women: a community study. *Am. J. Clin. Nutr. 41*:1045–1053.

Spittle, C. R. (1971). Atherosclerosis and vitamin C. *Lancet 2*:1280–1281.

Spittle, C. R. (1974). The action of vitamin C on blood vessels. *Am. Heart J. 88*:387–388.

Sram, R. J., Dobias, L., Pastorkova, A., Rossner, P., and Janca, L. (1983a). Effects of ascorbic acid prophylaxis on the frequency of chromosome aberrations in the peripheral lymphocytes of coal-tar workers. *Mutation Res. 120*:181–186.

Sram, R. J., Samkova, I., and Hola, N. (1983b). High-dose ascorbic acid prophylaxis in workers occupationally exposed to halogenated ethers. *J. Hyg. Epidemiol. Microbiol. Immunol. 27*:305–318.

Sram, R. J., Cerna, M., and Hola, N. (1986). Effect of ascorbic acid prophylaxis in groups occupationally exposed to mutagens. *Prog. Clin. Biol. Res. 209B*:327–335.

Stankova, L., Riddle, M., Larned, J., Burry, K., Menashe, D., Hart, J., and Bigley, R. (1984). Plasma ascorbate concentrations and blood cell dehydroascorbate transport in patients with diabetes mellitus. *Metabolism 33*:347–353.

Stevenson, N. R. (1974). Active transport of L-ascorbic acid in the human ileum. *Gastroenterology 67*:952–956.

Stich, H. F., Karim, J., Koropatnick, J., and Lo, L. (1976). Mutagenic action of ascorbic acid. *Nature 260*:722–724.

Sugimoto, T., Nakada, M., Fukase, M., Imai, Y., Kinoshita, Y., and Fujita, T. (1986). Effects of ascorbic acid on alkaline phosphatase activity and hormone responsiveness in the osteoblastic osteosarcoma cell line UMR-106. *Calcif. Tissue Int. 39*:171–174.

Sutor, D. J. and Johnston, C. S. (1988). Effect of a single, oral dose of vitamin C on interleukin-1 mediated host defense responses in men and women. *FASEB J 2*:A851.

Sutton, J. L., Basu, T. K., and Dickerson, J. W. T. (1983). Effect of large doses of ascorbic acid in man on some nitrogenous components of urine. *Hum. Nutr. Appl. Nutr. 37A*:136–140.

Tagliabue, A., Turconi, G., Allegrini, M., De Stefano, P., Borgna-Pignatti, C., Bongo, I., Dezza, L., and Cazzola, M. (1984). Ascorbic acid status in thalassemia major. *Haematologica* 69:542–547.

Tagliabue, A., Fiorentini, M., Rizzini, G., Turconi, G., and Cazzola, M. (1985). The effect of ascorbic acid supplementation on serum ferritin concentration in normal subjects. *Haematologica* 70:367–369.

Tappel, A. L. (1973). Lipid peroxidation damage to cell components. *Fed. Proc.* 32:1870–1874.

Taylor, A. (1989). Associations between nutrition and cataract. *Nutr. Rev.* 47:225–234.

Taylor, G. (1976). Vitamin C and stroke. *Lancet* 1:247.

Tebrock, H. E., Arminio, J. J., and Johnston, J. J. (1956). Usefulness of bioflavonoids and ascorbic acid in treatment of common cold. *J. Am. Med. Assoc.* 162:1227–33.

Thaete, L. G. and Grim, J. N. (1974). Fine structural effects of L-ascorbic acid on buccal epithelium. *Am. J. Clin. Nutr.* 27:719–727.

Tobian, L. (1988). Potassium and hypertension. *Nutr. Rev.* 46:273–283.

Trichopoulos, D., Ouranos, G., Day, N. E., Tzonou, A., Manousos, O., Papadimitriou, C., and Trichopoulos, A. (1985). Diet and cancer of the stomach: a case-control study in Greece. *Int. J. Cancer* 36:291–297.

Tsao, C. S., Miyashita, K., and Leung, P. Y. (1986). Effect of ascorbic acid on calcium elimination in humans. *J. Nutr. Sci. Vitaminol.* 32:437–446.

Tuyns, A. J. (1986). A case-control study on colorectal cancer in Belgium: preliminary results. *Sozial-Praventivmed.* 31:81–82.

Tuyns, A. J., Riboli, E., Doornbos, G., and Pequignot, G. (1987). Diet and esophageal cancer in Calvados (France). *Nutr. Cancer* 9:81–92.

Tyrell, D. A., Craig, J. W., Meada, T. W., and White, T. (1977). A trial of ascorbic acid in the treatment of the common cold. *Br. J. Prev. Soc. Med.* 31:189–91.

U. S. Department of Health and Human Services (1986). Detection and prevention of periodontal disease in diabetes. NIH Publication No. 86–1148.

Vallance, S. (1986). Platelets, leucocytes and buffy layer vitamin-C after surgery. *Hum. Nutr. Clin. Nutr.* 40C:35–41.

VanderJagt, D. J., Garry, P. J., and Bhagavan, H. N. (1987). Ascorbic acid intake and plasma levels in healthy elderly people. *Am. J. Clin. Nutr.* 45:290–294.

Varma, S. D., Chand, D., Sharma, Y. R., Kuck, J. F., and Richards, R. D. (1984). Oxidative stress on lens and cataract formation: role of light and oxygen. *Current Eye Res.* 3:35–57.

Verreault, R., Chu, J., Mandelson, M., and Shy, K. (1989). A case-control study of diet and invasive cervical cancer. *Int. J. Cancer 43*: 1050–1054.

Vollset, S. E. and Bjelke, E. (1983). Does consumption of fruit and vegetables protect against stroke? *Lancet 2*:742.

Wagner, D. A., Schultz, D. S., Deen, W. M., Young, V. R., and Tannenbaum, S. R. (1983). Metabolic fate of an oral dose of [15N]-labeled nitrate in humans: effect of diet supplementation with ascorbic acid. *Cancer Res. 43*:1921–1925.

Wagner, D. A., Shuker, D. E. G., Bilmazes, C., Obiedzinski, M., Baker, I., Young, V. R., and Tannenbaum, S. R. (1985). Effect of vitamins C and E on endogenous synthesis of N–nitrosamino acids in humans: precursor–product studies with [15N]nitrate. *Cancer Res. 45*:6519–6522.

Wahlberg, G. and Walldius, G. (1982). Lack of effect of ascorbic acid on serum lipoprotein concentrations in patients with hypertriglyceridaemia. *Atherosclerosis 43*:283–288.

Walker, G. H., Bynoe, M. L., and Tyrrell, D. A. (1967). Trial of ascorbic acid in prevention of colds. *Br. Med. J. 1*:603–6.

Wartanowicz, M., Panczenko-Kresowska, B., Ziemlanski, S., Kowalska, M., and Okolska, G. (1984). The effect of alpha-tocopherol and ascorbic acid on the serum lipid peroxide level in elderly people. *Ann. Nutr. Metab. 28*:186–191.

Wassertheil-Smoller, S., Romney, S. L., Wylie-Rosett, J., Slagle, S., Miller, G., Lucido, D., Duttagupta, C., and Palan, P. R. (1981). Dietary vitamin C and uterine cervical dysplasia. *Am. J. Epidemiol. 114*:714–724.

Weening, R. S., Schoorel, E. P., Roos, D., van Schaik, M. L. J., Voetman, A. A., Bot, A. A. M., Batenburg-Plenter, A. M., Willems, C., Zeijlemaker, W. P., and Astaldi, A. (1981). Effect of ascorbate on abnormal neutrophil, platelet, and lymphocyte function in a patient with the Chediak-Higashi syndrome. *Blood 57*:856–865.

Weitberg, A. B. and Weitzman, S. A. (1985). The effect of vitamin C on oxygen radical-induced sister-chromatid exchanges. *Mutation Res. 144*:23–26.

Wen-guang, W., Xue-cun, C., and Dong-sheng, L. (1986). Hematologic response to iron and ascorbic acid administration in preschool children with anemia. *Nutr. Res. 6*:241–248.

West, D. W., Slattery, M. L., Robison, L. M., Schuman, K. L., Ford, M. H., Mahoney, A. W., Lyon, J. L., and Sorensen, A. W. (1989). Dietary intake and colon cancer: sex- and antomic site-specific associations. *Am. J. Epidemiol. 130*:883–894.

Wilson, C. W. M. and Loh, H. S. (1973). Common cold and vitamin C. *Lancet 1*:638–641.

Wilson, C. W., Loh, H. S., and Foster, F. G. (1973). Common cold symptomatology and vitamin C. *Eur. J. Clin. Pharmacol.* 6:196– 202.

Winn, D. M., Ziegler, R. G., Pickle, L. W., Gridley, G., Blot, W. J., and Hoover, R. N. (1984). Diet in the etiology of oral and pharyngeal cancer among women from the southern United States. *Cancer Res.* 44:1216–1222.

Wu, A. H., Paganini-Hill, A., Ross, R. K., and Henderson, B. E. (1987). Alcohol, physical activity and other risk factors for colorectal cancer: a prospective study. *Br. J. Cancer* 55:687–694.

Yew, M-L. S. (1975). Biological variation in ascorbic acid needs. *Ann. NY Acad. Sci.* 258:451– 457.

Yoshioka, M., Matsushita, T., and Chuman, Y. (1984). Inverse association of serum ascorbic acid level and blood pressure or rate of hypertension in male adults aged 30–39 years. *Int. J. Vit. Nutr. Res.* 54:343–347.

You, W. C., Blot, W. J., Chang, Y. S., Ershow, A. G., Yang, Z. T., An, Q., Henderson, B., Xu, G. W., Fraumeni, J. F., and Wang, T. G. (1988). Diet and high risk of stomach cancer in Shandong, China. *Cancer Res.* 48:3518–3523.

Ziegler, R. G., Morris, L. E., Blot, W. J., Pottern, L. M., Hoover, R., and Fraumeni, J. F., Jr. (1981). Esophageal cancer among black men in Washington, DC. II. Role of nutrition. *J. Natl. Cancer Inst.* 67:1199–1206.

Ziemlanski, S., Panczenko-Kresowska, B., Warantowicz, M., and Klos, A. (1986). The effect of two-year supplementation with ascorbic acid and alpha-tocopherol on lipid, haematological and vitamin state in elderly women. *Zywienie Czlowieka Metabol.* 13:7–14.

7

Vitamin B₆

S. K. Gaby

I. INTRODUCTION

Vitamin B₆ (pyridoxine, pyridoxal, pyridoxamine, and the corresponding phosphorylated forms) is a water-soluble essential nutrient required for the metabolism of proteins, fats, and carbohydrates. The U.S. Recommended Daily Allowance (RDA) of vitamin B₆ is 2.0 mg. The best sources of the vitamin are fish, chicken, organ meats, eggs, and some grains and nuts. Because vitamin B₆ is required for amino acid metabolism, the need for the vitamin is related to protein intake. The natural forms of vitamin B₆ can be destroyed by heat processing, although pyridoxine hydrochloride, the form used in supplements and fortification, is quite stable. Dietary vitamin B₆ is converted to its active forms, pyridoxal-5'-phosphate (PLP) and pyridoxamine-5'-phosphate (PMP), in the liver, red blood cells, and other tissues of humans and animals.

Vitamin B₆ deficiency results in a variety of symptoms in humans, including poor growth, anemia, decreased immune response, convulsions, depression and confusion, skin lesions, and kidney stones. Vitamin B₆ deficiency has also been shown to cause atherosclerotic lesions in nonhuman primates (Rinehart and Greenberg, 1956).

Vitamin B₆ is not only involved in amino acid metabolism, but is also required for the production of neurotransmitters derived from amino acids, heme biosynthesis, purine biosynthesis, glycogen breakdown, and fatty acid and hormone metabolism.

II. HEALTH BENEFITS

A. Carpal Tunnel Syndrome

Nerve bundles pass through the carpal tunnel, a passageway at the wrist surrounded by dense ligaments. When the passage is narrowed, due to either inflammation, edema, or some other cause, there is a pressure on the median nerve, causing pain and/or numbness in the hands (carpal tunnel syndrome, CTS). This syndrome afflicts people who use their hands, wrists, or palms constantly, in repeated motions, such as assembly-line workers, typists, and keyboard operators. Treatment for CTS has involved the use of splints, antiinflammatory drugs, steroid injections, and surgery.

Ellis and co-workers (1977) reported that CTS patients were deficient in vitamin B_6, and that symptoms of the syndrome were relieved by vitamin B_6 supplements. A recent report corroborated the finding of low serum vitamin B_6 in CTS patients (Fuhr et al., 1989). Several studies, including a crossover placebo trial (Ellis et al., 1979), confirmed the efficacy of vitamin B_6 treatment (Ellis et al., 1981, 1982; Driskell, et al.; 1986, Ellis, 1987; Kasdan and Janes, 1987). Amadio found pyridoxine supplementation to be useful in mild cases of the syndrome (1985). No consistent improvement was reported, however, in a group of supplemented CTS patients with normal vitamin B_6 status (Smith et al., 1984). There was also no significant benefit from supplementation in a group of CTS subjects of unknown vitamin B_6 status enrolled in a recent double-blind study (Stransky et al., 1989). Byers et al., (1984) have proposed that the clinical improvement seen in some CTS patients after vitamin B_6 supplementation may be due to a correction of unrecognized peripheral neuropathy, which may compound the symptoms of CTS.

While subjects participating in these studies were frequently considered to have poor vitamin B_6 status, or even a deficiency by biochemical measures (Wolaniuk et al., 1983), none exhibited any of the classical vitamin B_6 deficiency symptoms. Also, supplementation with vitamin B_6 at levels of approximately 50–150 times U. S. RDA were required for optimal improvement. This may indicate that individuals with CTS have an unusually high metabolic demand for the vitamin or that the vitamin is active in some noncoenzyme role.

B. Premenstrual Syndrome

Premenstrual syndrome (PMS) is an ill-defined group of symptoms afflict-
ing a substantial proportion of women between the middle and the end
(luteal phase) of their menstrual cycles. Symptoms of PMS are varied and
numerous, including most commonly water retention, irritability, depression, tension, loss of coordination, and breast tenderness. Treatment is
often unsatisfactory and in many cases is directed at these individual
symptoms.

Decreased synthesis of neurotransmitters has been postulated to cause
the mood changes and water retention of PMS. A low serotonin level has
also been associated with increased appetite for carbohydrates and sleep
disturbances. Vitamin B6 is a required coenzyme in the synthesis of
serotonin and dopamine. Anxiety and fluid retention symptoms have been
correlated with the activity of aspartate aminotransferase, a vitamin
B6-dependent enzyme (Gallant et al., 1987); it was therefore suggested
that a decrease in active vitamin B6 may cause these PMS symptoms.
However, those symptoms most likely to be improved by neurotransmitter
normalization—depression and anxiety—have not been consistently reported to improve following vitamin B6 treatment (Kendall and Schnurr,
1987).

Although PMS sufferers have been shown to have normal blood levels of
vitamin B6 even during the luteal phase of their cycle (Ritchie and
Singkamani, 1986; van den Berg et al., 1986; Mira et al., 1988), there is
speculation that there may be a decrease in vitamin B6 entry into cells during PMS, due to cell transport (Brown et al., 1961)and enzyme binding
(Mason and Gullekson, 1960) competition from fluctuating hormone concentrations. According to such a model, an increase in vitamin B6 concentration could overcome competition and may explain the relief of symptoms seen in some women following high-dose vitamin B6 supplementation
(Barr, 1984). However, some workers have found no significant benefit
from vitamin B6 supplementation (Hagen et al., 1985; Smallwood et al.,
1986; Malmgren et al., 1987). Others report only a trend toward generalized improvement (Williams et al., 1985).

The studies that showed the greatest response to vitamin B6 treatment
used relatively high doses of the vitamin (up to 500 mg/day). However, a
good response has been reported at the relatively moderate dose of 50 mg/
day (25 times U.S. RDA) (Mattes and Martin, 1982).

The complexity of PMS and the subjective nature of symptom reporting
continue to result in controversy in the lay and scientific literature. Nonetheless, the current evidence indicates that vitamin B6 may be helpful in
alleviating some PMS symptoms.

C. Asthma

Low vitamin B6 (plasma pyridoxal-5'-phosphate) status has been reported in adult asthmatic subjects (Reynolds and Natta, 1985; Delport et al., 1988), though not in asthmatic children (Hall et al., 1982). This decrease in the active form of the vitamin may be due in part to the use of theophylline (a drug commonly used in the treatment of asthma) which lowers plasma PLP (Delport et al., 1988). Asthmatics may, however, have an altered metabolism of vitamin B6, suggested by the failure of high doses of the vitamin to increase blood PLP (Reynolds and Natta, 1985).

While vitamin B6 supplementation (50 mg twice a day) did not significantly increase plasma PLP in asthmatic subjects in one study, all supplemented subjects experienced a substantial decrease in the frequency and severity of asthma attacks (Reynolds and Natta, 1985). Similarly, a 200 mg/day dose of vitamin B6 to children with bronchial asthma significantly improved their condition and reduced their need for medication (Collipp et al., 1975). Clinical improvement was not significant at the 50 mg/day level.

The preliminary data on the use of vitamin B6 in the treatment of asthma are promising and justify further investigation.

D. Cardiovascular Health

In experimental animals, vitamin B6 deficiency causes atherosclerotic lesions similar to those seen in spontaneous human atherosclerosis (Rinehart and Greenberg, 1956).

Advanced atherosclerosis is also seen in children with homocystinuria, a genetic disorder. The metabolism of sulfur-containing amino acids is impaired in individuals with this disease, which may be due to a defect in the enzyme cystathionine synthase. This causes an accumulation of homocysteine. The metabolism of homocysteine to methionine involves three enzymes: a vitamin B6-, a folic acid-, and a vitamin B12- containing enzyme. Homocystinuria and/or homocystinemia can result from a defect in any of these enzymes, although the defect is most prevalent in the vitamin B6 enzyme. Homocysteine has been found to be highly atherogenic in animals (Linder, 1985) and may contribute to atherosclerosis in humans (McCully, 1969).

An increase in plasma homocysteine can also result from an inadequate intake of vitamin B6, as suggested by the fact that cystathionine synthase is vitamin B6-dependent. An epidemiological study compared the vitamin B6 intake and plasma homocysteine levels of men considered at high risk of coronary heart disease (on the basis of blood pressure and blood cholesterol levels) with those of men considered at low risk (Swift and Schultz, 1986). Mean dietary intake of vitamin B6 was 86% of the (1980) RDA in the low-risk group and 68% of the (1980) RDA in the high-risk group, although the difference was not statistically significant. Dietary vitamin B6 intake was negatively associated with protein-bound homocysteine levels, and men in the high-risk group had significantly higher plasma free homocysteine levels. This preliminary study suggests that marginally low vitamin B6 status may contribute to the development of coronary heart disease by increasing plasma homocysteine (Swift and Schultz, 1986).

The suggestion that vitamin B6 plays a role in cardiovascular health is consistent with epidemiological observations. Atherosclerosis is prevalent in developed countries where meat intake is high and diets are typically high in sulfur-containing amino acids and relatively low in vitamin B6 (Willett, 1985). (However, numerous other factors are significant in assessing these findings, such as the type of fat, cholesterol, and fiber intake.) Although vitamin B6 levels were not correlated with the incidence of ischemic heart disease in one study (Rossouw et al., 1985), low levels of plasma PLP were associated with two risk factors for coronary artery disease: smoking and increasing age (Serfontein et al., 1986).

Additional circumstantial evidence for an association between vitamin B6 and heart disease has been reported. For example, plasma pyridoxal-5'-phosphate levels were lower in individuals who had just had a myocardial infarction than in controls (Serfontein et al., 1985), although this may be an acute effect of the heart attack and not a causal factor (Vermaak et al., 1987).

A relationship between vitamin B6 status and cardiovascular health is suggested by data drawn from diverse areas of research and requires more extensive study.

E. Diabetic Neuropathy

Early studies showed that vitamin B6 deficiency caused neuropathology in monkeys (Victor and Adams, 1956). The peripheral neuropathy common in diabetics may also be associated with pyridoxine deficiency. Diabetics who experienced neuropathic symptoms, and whose urine contained tryptophan metabolites indicative of pyridoxine deficiency, were given 150 mg of vitamin B6 per day for 6 weeks (Jones and Gonzalez, 1978). The treatment eliminated symptoms of neuropathy in all subjects. In another group of diabetics with peripheral neuropathy given the same treatment for 4 months, symptoms were not improved significantly more then in the group receiving a placebo (Levin et al., 1981). However, only 1 of these 18 subjects had a low initial plasma PLP level. A recent, uncontrolled study indicated that 150 mg/day pyridoxine supplementation gradually improved pain scores in diabetics with painful neuropathy (Bernstein and Lobitz, 1988).

The most responsive period occurred between 12 and 16 weeks of supplementation, corresponding with a period of improved blood sugar control (Bernstein and Lobitz, 1988). Controlled double-blind trials are necessary to confirm the efficacy of pyridoxine supplementation in relieving painful diabetic neuropathies, and possibly improving control of blood glucose levels.

F. Immune Function

General malnutrition is known to have a deleterious effect on immune function. Frank vitamin B6 deficiency, whether primary or secondary, has also been shown to have a significant depressive effect on humoral and cellular immune system responses in humans and animals (Hodges et al., 1962; Beisel, 1982; Chandra and Puri, 1985; Bendich and Cohen, 1988).

Studies with mice suggest that very high dietary levels of vitamin B6 may significantly suppress induced tumor development (Gridley et al., 1987) and increase the cellular immune response (Gridley et al., 1988) in comparison with normal intake of the vitamin. However, another group reported that while typical dietary levels of vitamin B6 were necessary for normal immune response, excess quantities were of no additional value in the murine model (Ha et al., 1984).

Elderly people may have an increased requirement for vitamin B6 (Ribaya-Mercado et al., 1988). This same group tends to have a poor intake of the vitamin (Driskell, 1978), putting elderly people at risk for inadequate vitamin B6 status. A placebo-controlled trial was conducted with a small group of healthy elderly subjects given supplemental vitamin B6 (50 mg/day for 2 months) (Talbott et al., 1987). Before the trial, dietary intake of vitamin B6 by the subjects was approximately 75% of U.S. RDA. Supplementation was associated with significant increases in lymphocyte response to several mitogens. It would be interesting to evaluate the effects of vitamin B6 supplementation on in vivo measures of immune response in future studies in this area.

III. SAFETY

Large intakes of pyridoxine (2–6 g/day) have been associated with motor and sensory neuropathy (Schaumburg et al., 1983). These symptoms were noted in a case where an individual ingested 1.5 – 4.5 g vitamin B6 per day (Foca, 1985). Daily supplementation with 2 g of pyridoxine for 2 years was associated with reversible dermatosis and sensory neuropathy in one case (Friedman et al., 1986). Parry and Bredesen (1985) described neuropathies in a group of 16 self-supplementing individuals. Vitamin B6 dosages ranged from 200 mg to 5 g/day. One subject reported taking no more than 200 mg/day over a 3-year period, although most subjects were taking 2 g/day for at least 6 months when symptoms were noted (Parry and Bredesen, 1985). In an additional case report, supplementation with 1 g/day of vitamin B6 was associated with reversible sensory neuropathy (Waterston and Gilligan, 1987). In an uncontrolled study, neurological symptoms were associated with supplementation in women having average daily intakes as low as 117 mg/day for about 3 years (in comparison with asymptomatic women supplementing with an average 116 mg/day for about 1 1/2 years) (Dalton and Dalton, 1987).

A review of the published literature indicates that daily doses of vitamin B6 under 500 mg (250 times U.S. RDA) for up to 6 months appear to be safe (Cohen and Bendich, 1986).

Table 1 Summary of Research on the Benefits of Vitamin B6 Above U.S. RDA Level

Health condition	Current knowledge	Supplement
Carpal tunnel syndrome	8 studies reported a beneficial effect of supplementation; 2 studies found no consistent benefit	100–300 mg/day
Premenstrual syndrome	Vitamin B6 status does not differ between PMS sufferers and others, but supplementation appears to relieve some symptoms in some women	50–200 mg/day
Asthma	Significant benefit of supplemental B6 in relieving asthma reported in 2 studies	100–200 mg/day
Diabetic neuropathy	In 2 studies, supplements reduced pain; no effect in 1 study, where blood vitamin B6 levels were normal	150 mg/day
Immune function	Vitamin B6 deficiency associated with impaired immune function; supplements improved lymphocyte response to mitogens in elderly	50 mg/day

IV. SUMMARY

A summary of the research on the health benefits of vitamin B6 intake above the U.S. RDA level is presented in Table 1.

Vitamin B6 supplementation significantly reduces the symptoms of CTS in many patients. CTS may be associated with an increased demand for the vitamin.

Although the reports are controversial, vitamin B6 supplementation appears to relieve symptoms of PMS in some women.

There are some preliminary reports of relief of asthmatic symptoms with vitamin B6 supplementation.

Although mainly still speculative, a number of different observations suggest that a poor vitamin B6 status can be a factor in the causation of atherosclerosis.

Diabetic peripheral neuropathy may be associated with low vitamin B6 status. Vitamin B6 supplementation may relieve neuropathic symptoms.

Preliminary data, based mainly on animal studies, indicate that vitamin B6 may play a role in improving immune system functions.

Very high dose intakes of vitamin B6 have been associated with sensory and motor neuropathy. Daily intakes below 500 mg for up to 6 months, however, appear to be safe.

REFERENCES

Amadio, P. C. (1985). Pyridoxine as an adjunct in the treatment of carpal tunnel syndrome. *J. Hand Surg. 10*:237–241.

Barr, W. (1984). Pyridoxine supplements in the premenstrual syndrome. *Practitioner 228*:425–427.

Beisel, W. R. (1982). Single nutrients and immunity. *Am. J. Clin. Nutr. 35*:417–468.

Bendich, A. and Cohen, M. (1988). B vitamins: effects on specific and non-specific immune responses. In *Nutrition and Immunology*, R. K. Chandra (Ed.). Alan R. Liss, New York, pp. 101–123.

Bernstein, A. L. and Lobitz, C. S. (1988). A clinical and electrophysiologic study of the treatment of painful diabetic neuropathies with pyridoxine. In *Clinical and Physiological Applications of Vitamin B–6*, J. E. Leklem and R. D. Reynolds (Eds.). Alan R. Liss, New York, pp. 415–423.

Brown, R. R., Thornton, M. J., and Price, J. M. (1961). The effect of vitamin supplementation on the urinary excretion of tryptophan metabolites by pregnant women. *J. Clin. Invest. 40*:617–623.

Byers, C.M., DeLisa, J.A., Frankel, D.L., and Kraft, G.H. (1984). Pyridoxine metabolism in carpal tunnel syndrome with and without peripheral neuropathy. *Arch. Phys. Med. Rehabil. 65*:712–716.

Chandra, R. K. and Puri, S. (1985). Vitamin B–6 modulation of immune
responses and infection. In *Vitamin B–6: Its Role in Health and Disease*, R. D. Reynolds and J. E. Leklem (Eds.). Alan R. Liss, New York,
pp. 163–175.

Cohen, M. and Bendich, A. (1986). Safety of pyridoxine—a review of human and animal studies. *Toxicol. Lett. 34*:129–139.

Collipp, P .J., Goldzier, S., Weiss, N., Soleymani, Y., and Snyder, R. (1975).
Pyridoxine treatment of childhood bronchial asthma. *Ann. Allergy
35*:93–97.

Dalton, K. and Dalton, M. J. T. (1987). Characteristics of pyridoxine over-
dose neuropathy syndrome. *Acta. Neurol. Scand. 76*:8–11.

Delport, R., Ubbink, J. B., Serfontein, W. J., Becker, P. J., and Walters, L.
(1988). Vitamin B6 nutritional status in asthma: the effect of theophylline therapy on plasma pyridoxal–5′–phosphate and pyridoxal levels.
Int. J. Vit. Nutr. Res. 58:67–72.

Driskell, J. A. (1978). Vitamin B6 status of the elderly. In *Human Vitamin
B6 Requirements*, Committee on Dietary Allowances, Food and Nutrition Board, National Research Council, Washington, DC, pp. 252–256.

Driskell, J. A., Wesley, R. L., and Hess, I. E. (1986). Effectiveness of pyridoxine hydrochloride treatment on carpal tunnel syndrome patients.
Nutr. Rep. Int. 34:1031–1040.

Ellis, J. M. (1987). Treatment of carpal tunnel syndrome with vitamin B6.
Southern Med. J. 80:882–884.

Ellis, J. M., Azuma, J., Watanabe, T., Folkers, K., Lowell, J. R., Hurst, G.
A., Ahn, C. H., Shuford, E. H., Jr., and Ulrich, R. F. (1977). Survey and
new data on treatment with pyridoxine of patients having a clinical
syndrome including carpal tunnel and other defects. *Res. Commun.
Chem. Pathol. Pharmacol. 17*:165–177.

Ellis, J., Folkers, K., Watanabe, T., Kaji, M., Saji, S., Caldwell, J.W., Temple, C.A., and Wood, F.S. (1979). Clinical results of a cross-over treatment with pyridoxine and placebo of the carpal tunnel syndrome. *Am.
J. Clin. Nutr. 32*:2040–2046.

Ellis, J. M., Folkers, K., Levy, M., Takemura, K., Shizukuishi, S., Ulrich,
R., and Harrison, P. (1981). Therapy with vitamin B6 with and without
surgery for treatment of patients having the idiopathic carpal tunnel
syndrome. *Res. Commun. Chem. Pathol. Pharmacol. 33*:331–344.

Ellis, J. M., Folkers, K., Levy, M., Shizukuishi, S., Lewandowski, J., Nishii,
S., Schubert, H. A., and Ulrich, R. (1982). Response of vitamin B6 defi-

ciency and the carpal tunnel syndrome to pyridoxine. *Proc. Natl. Acad. Sci. USA* 79:7494–7498.

Foca, F.J. (1985). Motor and sensory neuropathy secondary to excessive pyridoxine ingestion. *Arch. Phys. Med. Rehabil.* 66:634–636.

Friedman, M. A., Resnick, J. S., and Baer, R. L.(1986). Subepidermal vesicular dermatosis and sensory peripheral neuropathy caused by pyridoxine abuse. *J. Am. Acad. Dermatol.* 14:915–917.

Fuhr, J. E., Farrow, A., and Nelson, H. S., Jr. (1989). Vitamin B6 levels in patients with carpal tunnel syndrome. *Arch. Surg.* 124:1329–1330.

Gallant, M. P., Bowering, J., Short, S. H., Turkki, P. R., and Badawy, S. (1987). Pyridoxine and magnesium status of women with premenstrual syndrome. *Nutr. Res.* 7:243–252.

Gridley, D. S., Shultz, T. D., Stickney, D. R., and Slater, J. M. (1988). In vivo and in vitro stimulation of cell-mediated immunity by vitamin B6. *Nutr. Res.* 8:201–207.

Gridley, D. S., Stickney, D. R., Nutter, R. L., Slater, J. M., and Shultz, T. D. (1987). Suppression of tumor growth and enhancement of immune status with high levels of dietary vitamin B6 in BALB/c mice. *J. Natl. Cancer Inst.* 78:951–959.

Ha, C., Miller, L. T., and Kerkvliet, N. I. (1984) The effect of vitamin B6 deficiency on cytotoxic immune responses of T cells, antibodies, and natural killer cells, and phagocytosis by macrophages. *Cell Immunol* 85:318–329.

Hagen, I., Nesheim, B. I., and Tuntland, T. (1985). No effect of vitamin B6 against premenstrual tension. *Acta Obstet. Gynecol. Scand.* 64: 667–670.

Hall, M. A., Thom, H., and Russell, G. (1982). Erythrocyte aspartate amino transferase activity in asthmatic and non-asthmatic children and its enhancement by vitamin B6. *Ann. Allergy* 47:464–466.

Hodges, R. E., Bean, W. B., Ohlson, M. A., and Bleiler, R. E. (1962). Factors affecting human antibody response. IV. Pyridoxine deficiency. *Am. J. Clin. Nutr.* 11:180–186.

Jones, C. L. and Gonzalez, V. (1978). Pyridoxine deficiency: a new factor in diabetic neuropathy. *J. Am. Podiatr. Assoc.* 68:646–653.

Kasdan, M. L. and Janes, C. (1987). Carpal tunnel syndrome and vitamin B6. *Plast. Reconstruct. Surg.* 79:456–459.

Kendall, K. E. and Schnurr, P. P. (1987). The effects of vitamin B6 supplementation on premenstrual symptoms. *Obstet. Gynecol.* 70:145–149.

Levin, E. R., Hanscom, T. A., Fisher, M., Lauvstad, W. A., Lui, A., Ryan, A., Glockner, D., and Levin, S. R. (1981). The influence of pyridoxine in diabetic peripheral neuropathy. *Diabetes Care* 4:606–609.

Linder, M. C. (1985). Nutrition and atherosclerosis. In *Nutritional Biochemistry and Metabolism with Clinical Applications*, M. C. Linder (Ed.), Elsevier, New York, pp. 331–346.

Malmgren, R., Collins, A., and Nilsson, C.G. (1987). Platelet serotonin uptake and effects of vitamin B6–treatment in premenstrual tension. *Neuropsychobiology 18*:83–88.

Mason, M. and Gullekson, E. H. (1960). Estrogen-enzyme interactions: inhibition and protection of kynurenine transaminase by the sulfate esters of diethylstilbestrol, estradiol, and estrone. *J. Biol. Chem. 235*: 1312–1316.

Mattes, J. A. and Martin, D. (1982). Pyridoxine in premenstrual depression. *Hum. Nutr. Appl. Nutr. 36A*:131–133.

McCully, K. S. (1969). Vascular pathology of homocysteinemia: implications for the pathogenesis of arteriosclerosis. *Am. J. Pathol. 56*: 111–128.

Mira, M., Stewart, P. M., and Abraham, S. F. (1988). Vitamin and trace element status in premenstrual syndrome. *Am. J. Clin. Nutr. 47*: 636–641.

Parry, G. J. and Bredesen, D. E. (1985). Sensory neuropathy with low-dose pyridoxine. *Neurology 35*:1466–1468.

Reynolds, R. D. and Natta, C. L. (1985). Depressed plasma pyridoxal phosphate concentrations in adult asthmatics. *Am. J. Clin. Nutr. 41*: 684–688.

Ribaya–Mercado, J. D., Russell, R. M., Sahyoun, N., Morrow, F. D., and Gershoff, S. N. (1988). Vitamin B6 requirements of the elderly. *FASEB J. 2*:A847.

Rinehart, J. F. and Greenberg, L. D. (1956). Vitamin B6 deficiency in the rhesus monkey with particular reference to the occurrence of atherosclerosis, dental caries, and hepatic cirrhosis. *Am. J. Clin. Nutr. 4*:318–325.

Ritchie, C. D. and Singkamani, R. (1986). Plasma pyridoxal 5'–phosphate in women with the premenstrual syndrome. *Hum. Nutr. Clin. Nutr. 40C*:75–80.

Rossouw, J. E., Labadarios, D., Jooste, P. L., and Shephard, G. S. (1985). Lack of a relationship between plasma pyridoxal phosphate levels and ischaemic heart disease. *S. Afr. Med. J. 67*:539–541.

Schaumburg, H., Kaplan, J., Windebank, A., Vick, N., Rasmus, S., Pleasure, D., and Brown, M. J. (1983). Sensory neuropathy from pyridoxine abuse: a new megavitamin syndrome. *N. Engl. J. Med. 309*:445–448.

Serfontein, W. J., Ubbink, J. B., De Villiers, L. S., Rapley, C. H., and Becker, P. J. (1985). Plasma pyridoxal–5'–phosphate level as risk index for coronary artery disease. *Atherosclerosis 55*:357–361.

Serfontein, W. J., Ubbink, J. B., De Villiers, L. S., and Becker, P. J. (1986). Depressed plasma pyridoxal–5′–phosphate levels in tobacco-smoking men. *Atherosclerosis 59*:341–346.

Smallwood, J., Ah-Kye, D., and Taylor, I. (1986). Vitamin B6 in the treatment of pre-menstrual mastalgia. *Br. J. Clin. Pract. 40*:532–533.

Smith, G. P., Rudge, P. J., and Peters, T. J. (1984). Biochemical studies of pyridoxal and pyridoxal phosphate status and therapeutic trial of pyridoxine in patients with carpal tunnel syndrome. *Ann. Neurol. 15*:104–107.

Stransky, M., Rubin, A., Lava, N. S., and Lazaro, R. P. (1989). Treatment of carpal tunnel syndrome with vitamin B6: a double-blind study. *South. Med. J. 82*:841–842.

Swift, M. E. and Shultz, T. D. (1986). Relationship of vitamins B6 and B12 to homocysteine levels: risk for coronary heart disease. *Nutr. Rep. Int. 34*:1–14.

Talbott, M. C., Miller, L. T., and Kerkvliet, N. I. (1987). Pyridoxine supplementation: effect on lymphocyte responses in elderly persons. *Am. J. Clin. Nutr. 46*:659–664.

van den Berg, H., Louwerse, E. S., Bruinse, H. W., Thissen, J. T. N. M., and Schrijver, J. (1986). Vitamin B6 status of women suffering from premenstrual syndrome. *Hum. Nutr. Clin. Nutr. 40C*:441–450.

Vermaak, W. J. H., Barnard, H. C., Potgieter, G. M. and Theron, H. du T. (1987). Vitamin B6 and coronary artery disease: epidemiological observations and case studies. *Atherosclerosis 63*:235–238.

Victor, M. and Adams, R. D. (1956). The neuropathy of experimental vitamin B6 deficiency in monkeys. *Am. J. Clin. Nutr. 4*:346–353.

Waterston, J. A. and Gilligan, B. S. (1987). Pyridoxine neuropathy. *Med. J. Aust. 146*:640–642.

Willett, W. C. (1985). Does low vitamin B6 intake increase the risk of coronary heart disease? In *Vitamin B6: Its Role in Health and Disease*, R. D. Reynolds and J. E. Leklem, (Eds.). Alan R. Liss, New York, pp. 337–346.

Williams, M. J., Harris, R. I., and Dean, B. C. (1985). Controlled trial of pyridoxine in the premenstrual syndrome. *J. Int. Med. Res. 13*: 174–179.

Wolaniuk, A., Vadhanavikit, S., and Folkers, K. (1983). Electromyographic data differentiate patients with the carpal tunnel syndrome when double blindly treated with pyridoxine and placebo. *Res. Commun. Chem. Pathol. Pharmacol 41*:501–511.

8

Folic Acid

S.K. Gaby and A. Bendich

I. INTRODUCTION

Folic acid (pteroylglutamic acid) is a water-soluble essential nutrient. The U. S. recommended daily dietary allowance (RDA) of folic acid for adults is 400 µg; the U.S. RDA for pregnant women is 800 µg. Good food sources of folate are fresh leafy vegetables and fruit, yeast, and liver.

Folic acid is a precursor of several important enzyme cofactors required for the synthesis of nucleic acids and the metabolism of some amino acids. Insufficient intake of folic acid results in an inability to produce deoxyribonucleic acid (DNA), ribonucleic acid (RNA) and certain proteins. Without DNA replication and adequate protein synthesis, cell growth is arrested. A deficiency of folic acid may result in localized or end-organ deficiencies in tissues with rapid turnover, such as those of the uterine cervix (Whitehead et al., 1973; Butterworth et al., 1982), lungs (Heimberger et al., 1987), gastrointestinal tract (Lashner et al., 1989), and gums (Pack and Thompson, 1980). It has been proposed that gingival disease may respond to local folate repletion (Pack and Thomson, 1980; Pack, 1984,1986). Anemia is a common manifestation of folate deficiency owing to rapid red blood cell turnover and the high metabolic requirements of hematopoietic tissue.

A number of population groups in the United States are at risk for developing folate deficiency (Anderson and Talbot, 1981). The risk is high during growth phases and is therefore greatest in newborn infants (Anderson and Talbot, 1981), pregnant women (Colman et al., 1974; Huber et al., 1988), and adolescents (Bailey et al., 1984) especially females (Clark et al., 1987) and black and Hispanic adolescents in low income households (Bailey et al., 1982). According to NHANES II data, women aged 20–44 years are at greatest risk for folate deficiency (Senti and Pilch, 1985). A survey of the folate intake of a group of young children found that intake failed to meet recommended levels in any socioeconomic subgroup (Martinez, 1982). Low dietary intake of folic acid is also typical of the elderly, in whom poor folic acid status is common (Bates et al., 1980). In addition, some forms of dietary folic acid may be less well absorbed by elderly than by younger individuals although the form of the vitamin in supplements is well absorbed (Baker et al., 1978). The use of some drugs, including alcohol, and deficiencies of other nutrients can also have deleterious effects on folic acid status (Anderson and Talbot, 1981).

II. BIRTH DEFECTS

A. Folic Acid During Pregnancy

There is an increased requirement for folic acid during pregnancy, owing to the substantial increase in maternal hematopoiesis and growth of the conceptus. In addition, investigators have documented a high rate of catabolism of folic acid during pregnancy in animals and humans (Courtney et al., 1987).

B. Neural Tube Defects

A deficiency of folic acid early in a pregnancy, before closure of the neural tube (the tissue that becomes the brain and spinal cord), may be causally related to neural tube defects (NTD) (Laurence et al., 1981; Smithells et al., 1976, 1980). NTD include anencephaly, spina bifida, and encephalocele. In the United States, NTD occur in about 1.7 births per thousand (Zackai et al., 1978).

A linear relationship was found between red blood cell folate level and the number of previous pregnancies resulting in neural tube defects, with the lowest folate levels in women having a history of three or four such pregnancies (Yates et al., 1987). Yates et al. (1987) suggest that certain individuals may have a defect in folate metabolism, since a given level of dietary folate failed to cause the same red blood cell folate increase in those with NTD pregnancies as in controls. Also, the dietary folate intake of women of reproductive age is likely to be low (Daniel et al., 1971) and serum folate levels drop steadily during gestation (Hall et al., 1976).

1. Studies of Serum Folate Levels and Diet

Folic acid deficiency has been well documented as a cause of congenital malformations in animals (for a review see Briggs, 1976). A casual relationship between folate deficiency and birth defects has also been postulated in humans (Laurence et al., 1981). However, few placebo-controlled intervention trials have been done. Epidemiological studies have shown associations between low serum levels of folate and low dietary intake, and adverse pregnancy outcomes.

A small group of women with NTD-affected pregnancies were found to have significantly lower folate levels in their red blood cells and lower vitamin C in their white blood cells during the first trimester of pregnancy than women who delivered normal infants (Smithells et al., 1976). However, other investigators found no significant differences in serum folic acid levels in mothers of NTD infants compared with control mothers (Hall 1972; Molloy et al., 1985). This suggests that serum folate level alone may not be directly related to the risk for NTD in pregnancy, whereas red blood cell folate, an indicator of long-term folate status, may be more predictive. An intervention study of high-risk women with a previous NTD pregnancy and low-risk groups showed a similar trend: low blood concentrations of folic acid, riboflavin, and vitamin C were found in the high-risk subjects; these low levels were improved by vitamin supplements (Schorah et al., 1983).

A recent study found that dietary intake of free (supplemental) folate during the first 6 weeks of pregnancy was inversely related to the risk of NTD pregnancy (Bower and Stanley, 1989). Total (dietary and supplemental) folate was less strongly associated with reduced risk. Total folic acid intakes in the highest quartile were associated with a greater than 60% lowered risk of NTD, relative to the lowest quartile. The risk was reduced by 80% among those with the highest intake of free folate (Bower and Stanley, 1989).

A cohort of 22,776 pregnant women responded to an extensive questionnaire concerning factors that may be related to pregnancy outcome, including vitamin use (Milunsky et al., 1989). The prevalence of NTD among infants of those using folic acid-containing multivitamins during the first 6 weeks of pregnancy was 0.9 per 1000. Among those who did not use a vitamin supplement during that time, the prevalence of NTD affected pregnancies was 3.5 per 1000. The 60% reduction in risk was highly significant. An even greater risk reduction was seen in individuals at greater risk for NTD pregnancies based on family histories (13.0/1000 unsupplemented vs. 3.5/1000 supplemented). Supplementation begun after the seventh week of pregnancy or the use of multivitamins without folic acid was not associated with a reduced incidence of NTD.

2. NTD: Clinical Intervention

In Britain, women who have carried a fetus with an NTD have a 5% risk of having another child with the same defect in a subsequent pregnancy (Wynn, 1982). The effect of vitamin supplementation on the risk of having a second infant with an NTD was studied in a group of 324 women (Smithells et al., 1980). The women received a multivitamin-mineral supplement which included 360 µg folic acid, 4000 IU vitamin A, 40 mg vitamin C, and 1.5 mg riboflavin. The control subjects either became pregnant before the trial or refused supplementation. Of the 178 infants/fetuses of the fully supplemented women, one suffered an NTD (0.6%). There were 13 cases of NTD recurrence among the 260 infants/fetuses carried by unsupplemented women (5.0%). This highly statistically significant result was repeated in a second similar trial (Smithells et al., 1983) (Table 1).

Another study, which was initiated as a placebo-controlled intervention trial aimed at preventing recurrence of NTD, was conducted in 44 pregnant women given a 4 mg daily supplement of folic acid (Laurence et al., 1981). An additional 16 women received supplements, but did not take them as instructed, and 51 received placebos. The subjects' diets were classified as good, fair, or inadequate. There was no reappearance of NTD in the pregnancy outcomes of supplemented mothers. Among those who did not comply with the treatment schedule there were 2 cases of NTD, and there were 4 cases among the pregnancies with no vitamin supplementation. The complete lack of recurrence of NTD in pregnancies of the fully supplemented group (0%) was significantly lower than the recurrence in the noncompliant and unsupplemented groups considered together (9%). However, the practice of considering non-compliers as controls has been questioned (Mamtani and Watkins, 1981). All six infants with NTD were born to women with inadequate diets, and the influence of diet was highly significant.

A reduction in the incidence of NTD recurrence was also seen when pregnant women moved from a poor diet to a nutritionally adequate diet (Laurence, 1983).

3. NTD and Medication During Pregnancy

In contrast to studies done on the serum of nonmedicated NTD mothers and controls, serum folate level was related to outcome in 47 pregnancies during which anticonvulsants were administered to control maternal epilepsy (Dansky et al., 1987). Anticonvulsants, such as phenytoin, tend to interfere with the normal metabolism of folic acid. The risk of an unsuccessful pregnancy or birth defect was 11.8% in women with a serum folate

TABLE 1 Summary of Studies on Folic Acid Supplementation and Birth Defects

Number of pregnancies	Supplementation	Birth defect	Recurrence (%)	Reference
178	Multivitamin/mineral (0.36 mg. folic acid)	NTD	0.6	Smithells et al.,1980
260	None	NTD	5.0[a]	Smithells et al.,1983
254	Multivitamin/mineral	NTD	0.9	
64	Partial use of multivitamin/mineral	NTD	0	
219	None	NTD	5.1[a]	Laurence et al., 1981
44	4 mg folic acid	NTD	0	
16	Partial use of folic acid	NTD	12.5 } 8.9	
51	None	NTD	7.8[a]	Conway, 1958
59	Multivitamins with 0.5 mg folic acid	Cleft palate/lip	0	
78	None	Cleft palate/lip	5.1	
228	5 mg folic acid, 10 mg B6, stress formula vitamin	Cleft palate/lip	3.1	Briggs, 1976
417	None	Cleft palate/lip	4.8	
228	5 mg folic acid, 10 mg B6, stress formula vitamin	Cleft lip	1.5	Briggs, 1976
417	None	Cleft lip	4.1	

[a]Statistically significant difference from treatment.

level of 4 ng/ml or higher; the risk rose to 46.2% with lower serum folate levels.

A retrospective study found that among 66 births to women taking a folate-antagonizing anticonvulsive drug for epilepsy, 15% of the infants had congenital malformations including NTD (Biale and Lewenthal, 1984). This group served as the control for an intervention trial. When folic acid supplements (2.5–5 mg/day) were given with the drug during another 33 pregnancies, all infants were born alive, had normal body weights, and no birth defects were seen.

C.   Cleft Palate/Cleft Lip: Clinical Intervention

Citing animal data showing a positive association between nutritional deficiencies and the incidence of cleft lip/cleft palate, Conway (1958) gave vitamin supplements to women who had previously given birth to an infant with these malformations. The supplement included the water soluble vitamins, with 500 μg of folic acid, and vitamins A and D. Vitamin supplementation was administered in a daily capsule and by injection every other day during the first 3 months of 59 pregnancies in 39 women. No recurrence of cleft palate/lip was seen (0%). Forty-eight other women received no vitamins during 78 subsequent pregnancies, and there were four recurrences of cleft lip and/or cleft palate (5.1%)

Over a 19–year period, 645 women who had had a child with cleft palate and/or cleft lip were studied through a plastic surgery practice (Briggs, 1976). These women were advised to take a vitamin supplement during any future pregnancy. The supplement consisted of 5 mg folic acid, 10 mg pyridoxine hydrochloride (B6), and a stress formula vitamin (10 mg thiamine, 10 mg riboflavin, 100 mg niacinamide, 300 mg vitamin C, 2 mg vitamin B6, 4 μg vitamin B12, and 20 mg calcium pantothenate). These supplements were recommended as a daily dose to be taken from the time of the first "suspicion" of pregnancy to at least the fifth month. During subsequent pregnancies, 417 women took no vitamin supplement, and the incidence of cleft palate and/or cleft lip was 4.8%. Of the 228 women who took the vitamins in the first trimester and/or before conception, the recurrence of cleft palate/lip was 3.1%. Cleft lip (in combination with cleft palate or alone) recurred in 4.1% of the non-supplement users' infants, compared with 1.5% of all subsequent births to the vitamin-supplemented mothers. The differences were not statistically significant.

III.   DYSPLASIA

Abnormal cytological changes are characteristic of some precancerous conditions. Poor folic acid status has been associated with megaloblastic changes in the cells of the uterine cervix (Whitehead et al., 1973) and intestinal epithelium (Bianchi et al., 1970). Additionally, dysplasia of the cervicovaginal epithelium appeared in folate-deficient monkeys (Mohanty and Das, 1982). These findings suggest that folic acid status may be causally related to the development of dysplasia and, subsequently, cancer. A significantly lower level of plasma folate has been reported in cases of existing cervical cancer compared with controls (Orr et al., 1985).

As noted above, folic acid is important for normal nucleic acid synthesis . An inadequate supply of folate may affect dysplasia by impeding DNA repair and potentiating mutation. Moderate folate depletion has been associated with an increased appearance of chromosomal damage in blood cells; this increase can be normalized with folic acid supplementation (Everson et al., 1988). It has been suggested that localized folate deficiency may occur in certain tissues, and that deficient cells become more susceptible to chromosomal damage and cancerous growth (Whitehead et al., 1973; Heimburger et al., 1987). Abnormal cervical cells ("folic acid deficiency cells") have been reported in women with folic acid deficiency anemia; such cells disappear within days following folic acid supplementation (Ritter et al., 1973). In cervical cancer, which is associated with human papillomavirus in at least 90% of the cases (Kurman et al., 1988), poor folate status may facilitate the incorporation of viral genetic material into the host cell. Although this mechanism is speculative at present, a methyl-deficient diet has been associated with increased incorporation of viral RNA into mouse liver cells (Hsieh et al., 1989).

A. Cervical Dysplasia and Oral Contraceptives

The use of hormonal contraceptives appears to influence folate status and signs of cervical dysplasia. Low levels of folate were found in megaloblastic cervicovaginal cells of women taking oral contraceptive agents; the cellular abnormalities resolved or improved substantially in response to folic acid supplementation (10mg/day × 3 weeks) (Whitehead et al., 1973). A summary of early reports concluded that approximately one-fifth of oral contraceptive users had megaloblastic changes in the cervicovaginal epithelium that were completely reversed by folic acid supplementation (Lindenbaum et al., 1975).

Butterworth and others measured red blood cell folate concentration and assigned biopsy scores to 47 cervical dysplasia patients and controls (Butterworth et al., 1982). Initially, folate concentrations were lower in oral contraceptive users than nonusers, and lowest in users with dysplasia. After a double-blind, 3–month placebo–controlled trial, using 10 mg folic acid, treated subjects had significantly better biopsy scores than controls.

B. Bronchial Squamous Metaplasia

Abnormalities in bronchopulmonary cells are often seen preceding lung cancer. Lowered plasma and red blood cell folic acid levels have been associated with bronchial metaplasia in smokers (Heimburger et al., 1985). A preliminary trial in smokers with precancerous lesions of the lung indicates that folate supplementation may be useful in the treatment of this type of dysplasia (Heimburger et al., 1988). Seventy-three men with a history of smoking at least one pack of cigarettes per day for at least 20 years were given either a placebo or 10 mg folate with 500μg vitamin B_{12} for 4 months. The treated group showed a significant reduction in irregular bronchial squamous cells (Heimburger et al., 1988).

C. Ulcerative Colitis and Dysplasia

Chronic ulcerative colitis is associated with an increased incidence of dysplasia and colon cancer. Folic acid supplements were given to 99 individuals with ulcerative colitis, and the development of dysplasia or cancer was monitored (Lashner et al., 1989). Folic acid supplementation (either 1 mg tablets or 0.4 mg as part of a multivitamin supplement) was associated with a 62% reduction in the incidence of neoplasia. This relationship remained after adjusting for potential confounders, although the association was not statistically significant at the 95% confidence interval. While this trial is preliminary, the findings are intriguing. In light of other data on folate status and precancerous lesions, follow-up studies are warranted.

IV. CARDIOVASCULAR HEALTH

Folic acid is required for the conversion of homocysteine to methionine, and a deficiency of the vitamin is associated with homocystinemia. High circulating homocysteine levels are a risk factor for atherosclerosis (McCully, 1969; see Chapter 7, "Vitamin B_6"). A strong inverse correlation was found between serum folate and homocysteine levels in subjects with higher than normal homocysteine levels (Kang et al., 1987).

High circulating levels of homocysteine were found in a group of postmenopausal women with normal serum and red cell folate levels. Folic acid supplementation (5 mg/day for 4 weeks) lowered homocysteine levels in this group (Brattstrom et al., 1985). Brattstrom et al. (1988) found that normal subjects given 5 mg/day of folic acid for 2 weeks had a significant decrease in circulating homocysteine levels. The decrease was most dramatic in individuals with initially high homocysteine levels.

V. SAFETY

Folic acid is generally considered to be safe even at very high levels of intake (Preuss, 1978; Butterworth and Tamura,1989). Some gastrointestinal upset and an altered sleep pattern have been reported at doses of 15 mg/day (Hunter et al., 1970), although this effect was not replicated (Hellstrom, 1971). It has also been reported that high-dose folic acid supplementation may interfere with zinc absorption (Wilson et al., 1983; Milne et al., 1984), but other recent studies have found that high-dose folic acid supplementation does not adversely effect zinc status (Keating et al., 1987; Butterworth et al., 1988; Krebs et al., 1988). A moderate intake of folic acid may cause a false negative result in screening for the X chromosome fragile site, a marker for mental retardation (Froster-Iskenius et al., 1987). A high intake of folic acid can also mask the clinical signs of pernicious anemia, and for that reason levels of the vitamin in supplements are regulated by the Food and Drug Administration through a food additive regulation.

VI. SUMMARY

Folic acid and multivitamin supplement use are associated with decreased recurrence of neural tube defects and cleft palate/cleft lip. Low maternal serum folate levels were associated with a substantially greater incidence of birth defects in infants whose mothers were taking anticonvulsant medication.

Subjects with cervical dysplasia were found to have lower serum folate levels than controls; supplementation with folic acid improved cytology scores of cases. Supplementation with folic acid also reduced the number of abnormal cells in cases of bronchial squamous metaplasia in smokers and lowered the incidence of neoplasia in chronic ulcerative colitis.

Preliminary findings suggest that folic acid may reduce cardiovascular disease by lowering homocysteine levels.

Folic acid is believed to be safe in normal subjects even at intakes as high as 15 mg/day.

REFERENCES

Anderson, S. A. and Talbot, J. M. (1981). A review of folate intake, methodology, and status. FDA technical report FDA/RF–82/13, Washington, DC.

Bailey, L. B., Wagner, P. A., Christakis, G. J., Davis, C. G., Appledorf, H., Araujo, P. E., Dorsey, E., and Dinning, J. S. (1982). Folacin and iron status and hematological findings in black and Spanish–American adolescents from urban low–income households. *Am. J. Clin. Nutr.* *35*:1023–1032.

Bailey, L. B., Wagner, P. A., Davis, C. G., and Dinning, J. S. (1984). Food frequency related to folacin status in adolescents. *J. Am. Diet. Assoc.* *84*:801–804.

Baker, H., Jaslow, S. P., and Frank, O. (1978). Severe impairment of dietary folate utilization in the elderly. *J. Am. Geriatr. Soc. 26:* 218–221.

Bates, C. J., Fleming, M., Paul, A. A., Black, A. E., and Mandal, A. R. (1980). Folate status and its relation to vitamin C in healthy elderly men and women. *Age Ageing 9*:241–248.

Biale, Y. and Lewenthal, H. (1984). Effect of folic acid supplementation on congenital malformations due to anticonvulsive drugs. *Eur. J. Obstet. Gynecol. Reprod. Biol. 18*:211–216.

Bianchi, A., Chipman, D. W., Dreskin, A., and Rosensweig, N. S. (1970). Nutritional folic acid deficiency with megaloblastic changes in the small bowel epithelium. *N. Engl. J. Med. 282*:859–861.

Bower, C. and Stanley, F. J. (1989). Dietary folate as a risk factor for neural-tube defects: evidence from a case-control study in Western Australia. *Med. J. Aust. 150*:613–619.

Brattstrom, L. E., Hultberg, B. L., and Hardebo, J. E., (1985). Folic acid responsive postmenopausal homocysteinemia. *Metabolism 34*: 1073–1077.

Brattstrom, L. E., Israelsson, B., Jeppsson, J. O., and Hultberg, B. L. (1988). Folic acid—an innocuous means to reduce plasma homocysteine. *Scand. J. Clin. Lab. Invest. 48*:215–221.

Briggs, R. M. (1976). Vitamin supplementation as a possible factor in the incidence of cleft lip/palate deformities in humans. *Clin. Plast. Surg. 3*:647–652.

Butterworth, C.E. and Tamura, T. (1989). Folic acid safety and toxicity. *Am. J. Clin. Nutr. 50*:353–358.

Butterworth, C. E., Hatch, K. D., Gore, H., Mueller, H., and Krumdieck, C. L. (1982). Improvement in cervical dysplasia associated with folic acid therapy in users of oral contraceptives. *Am. J. Clin. Nutr. 35*:73–82.

Butterworth, C. E., Hatch, K., Cole, P., Sauberlich, H. E., Tamura, T., Cornwell, P. E., and Soong, S. J. (1988). Zinc concentration in plasma and erythrocytes of subjects receiving folic acid supplementation. *Am. J. Clin. Nutr. 47*:484–486.

Clark, A. J., Mossholder, S., and Gates, R. (1987). Folacin status in adolescent females. *Am. J. Clin. Nutr. 46*:302–306.

Colman, N., Barker, M., Green, R., and Metz, J. (1974). Prevention of folate deficiency in pregnancy by food fortification. *Am. J. Clin. Nutr.* 27:339–344.

Conway, H. (1958). Effect of supplemental vitamin therapy on the limitation of incidence of cleft lip and cleft palate in humans. *Plast. Reconstruct. Surg.* 22:450–453.

Courtney, M. G., McPartlin, J. M., McNulty, H. M., Scott, J. M., and Weir, D. G. (1987). The cause of folate deficiency in pregnancy is increased catabolism of the vitamin. *Gastroenterology* 92:1355.

Daniel, W. A, Jr., Mounger, J. R., and Perkins, J. C. 1971. Obstetric and fetal complications in folate-deficient adolescent girls. *Am. J. Obstet. Gynecol.* 111:233–238.

Dansky, L. V., Andermann, E., Rosenblatt, D., Sherwin, A. L., and Andermann, F. (1987). Anticonvulsants, folate levels, and pregnancy outcome: a prospective study. *Ann. Neurol.* 21:176–182.

Everson, R. B., Wehr, C. M., Erexson, G. L., and MacGregor, J. T. (1988). Association of marginal folate depletion with increased human chromosomal damage in vivo: demonstration by analysis of micronucleated erythrocytes. *J. Natl. Cancer Inst.* 80:525–529.

Froster-Iskenius, U., Hall, J. G., and Curry, C. J.R. (1987). False negative results in patients with fra(X)(q) mental retardation taking oral vitamin supplements. *N. Engl. J. Med.* 316:1093.

Hall, M. H. (1972). Folic acid deficiency and congenital malformation. *J. Obstet. Gynaecol. Br. Commonw.* 79:159–161.

Hall, M. H., Pirani, B. B. K., and Campbell, D. (1976). The cause of the fall in serum folate in normal pregnancy. *Br. J. Obstet. Gynaecol.* 83:132–136.

Heimburger, D. C., Alexander, C. B., Birch, R., Butterworth, C. E., Bailey, W. C., and Krumdieck, C. L. (1988). Improvement in bronchial squamous metaplasia in smokers treated with folate and vitamin B_{12}: report of a preliminary randomized, double-blind intervention trial. *J. Am. Med. Assoc.* 259:1525–1530.

Heimburger, D. C., Bailey, W. C., Alexander, C. B., Birch, R., Combs, B., Soto, P., Saxon, D., Schnaper, H., and Krumdieck, C. L. (1985). Bronchial metaplasia in smokers associated with decreased folic acid levels. *Am. Rev. Respir. Dis.* 131:A392.

Heimburger, D. C., Krumdieck, C. L. and Butterworth, C. E. (1987). Role of folate in prevention of cancers of the lung and cervix. *J. Am. Coll. Nutr.* 6:425.

Hellstrom, L. (1971). Lack of toxicity of folic acid given in pharmacological doses to healthy volunteers. *Lancet* 1:59–61.

of neural-tube defects by periconceptional vitamin supplementation. *Lancet 1*:339–342.

Smithells, R. W., Seller, M. J., Harris, R., Fielding, D. W., Schorah, C. J., Nevin, N. C., Sheppard, S., Read, A. P., Walker, S., and Wild, J. (1983). Further experience of vitamin supplementation for prevention of neural tube defect recurrences. *Lancet 1*:1027–1031.

Whitehead, N., Reyner, F., and Lindenbaum, J. (1973). Megaloblastic changes in the cervical epithelium: an association with oral contraceptive therapy and reversal with folic acid. *J. Am. Med. Assoc. 226*:1421–1424.

Wilson, P. C., Greene, H. L., Murrell, J. E., and Ghishan, F. K. (1983). The effect of folic acid on the intestinal absorption of zinc. *Clin. Res. 31*:760A.

Wynn, J. (1982). Spina bifida: trials ahead. *Nature 299*:198.

Yates, J. R.W., Ferguson-Smith, M. A., Shenkin, A.,Guzman-Rodriguez, R., White, M., and Clark, B. J. 1987. Is disordered folate metabolism the basis for the genetic predisposition to neural tube defects? *Clin. Genet. 31:* 279–287.

Zackai, E. H., Spielman, R. S., Mellman, W. J., Ames, M., and Bodurtha, J. (1978). The risk of neural tube defects to first cousins of affected individuals. In *Prevention of Neural Tube Defects: The Role of alpha-Fetoprotein,* B. F. Crandall and M. A. B. Brazier (Eds.). Academic Press, New York, pp. 99–102.

9

Niacin

S. K. Gaby

I. INTRODUCTION

Niacin is a water-soluble essential nutrient available in relatively large amounts from meat and some nuts. Niacin in many foods (such as grains) is bound to other substances and therefore nutritionally unavailable (Darby et al., 1975). Niacin (nicotinic acid and nicotinamide) is a critical cofactor in numerous biochemical processes, notably energy metabolism. Niacin deficiency causes pellagra, a disease whose symptoms include dermatosis, oral lesions, anemia, diarrhea, and neurological abnormalities. The U.S. Recommended Daily Allowance for niacin for adults is 20 mg. A small proportion of dietary tryptophan (an essential amino acid) is converted to niacin in humans and most animals.

II. CARDIOVASCULAR DISEASE

High doses of niacin, as nicotinic acid, have been shown to be useful in the treatment of hyperlipidemia, since it reduces so-called "bad" cholesterol (low density lipoprotein cholesterol, LDL–C) and increases "good" cholesterol (high density lipoprotein cholesterol, HDL–C) (Yovos et al., 1982; Lees and Lees, 1984; Schaefer and Levy, 1985; Hoeg et al., 1986; Naito, 1987; Tikkanen and Nikkila, 1987). In a study comparing niacin with other coronary drugs in men who had had a heart attack, 15–year follow-up (9 years after treatment ended) showed an 11% lower mortality rate in the group receiving niacin, compared with the placebo group (Canner et al., 1986). No other treatment resulted in significantly lower mortality.

Unlike other agents used in the treatment of high blood lipids, niacin appears to block the initial synthesis and secretion of the LDL precursor, rather than removing LDL–C after it is already present (Hoeg et al., 1986; Perry, 1986). This is consistent with the earlier discovery that niacin has antilipolytic properties and therefore reduces the release of lipids into the bloodstream (Carlson and Oro, 1962). However, the exact mechanism by which niacin improves blood lipid profiles and cardiovascular health is not definitively known. It has been suggested that niacin reduces the catabolism of HDL (Shepherd et al., 1979). Niacin may also favorably alter the synthesis of arachidonic acid metabolites (Pattison et al., 1987), a potentially important factor in the development of atherosclerosis.

Nicotinic acid will stimulate histamine release and cause a temporary vasodilation, resulting in unpleasant symptoms of flushing associated with doses of about 75 mg or more. If levels are increased gradually, hyperlipidemic patients can often increase their tolerance to nicotinic acid. The quantity of nicotinic acid generally recommended for lowering cholesterol and triglycerides is in the range of 1.5 – 6 g/day (Naito, 1987). The vitamin appears to show a good dose-response lipid–lowering effect (Walldius and Wahlberg,1985).

Highly successful treatment for hyperlipidemia has been reported for nicotinic acid in combination with other drugs. Significant improvement, and in some cases a normalization of plasma cholesterol and LDL, was reported in patients with heterozygous familial hypercholesterolemia (an inherited hyperlipidemia) after treatment with niacin plus the cholesterol-lowering drug cholestyramine (Angelin et al., 1986). Use of a closely related drug, colestipol, administered with 3–12 g niacin per day led to an improvement in the lipid profiles of patients who had had coronary bypass surgery (and in some subjects, there was a measurable reduction in the degree of atherosclerosis) (Blankenhorn et al., 1987). Because nicotinic acid causes an increase in blood sugar (Shansky, 1981), niacin treatment is generally contraindicated in diabetics. However, a case report of diabetes mellitus with severe hypertriglyceridemia showed complete normalization of lipid values following combination treatment with insulin and 1.2 g/day nicotinic acid (Smith, 1981).

III. SAFETY

The majority of people who ingest large doses of nicotinic acid will feel skin flushing (Weiner et al., 1958). Most individuals will experience flushing with intakes as low as 50–100 mg. This reaction is not adverse and lasts about 20 minutes. About half of those taking the vitamin will develop a tolerance to this effect. The niacinamide form usually found in vitamin supplements does not cause this reaction (Bures, 1980), but neither does it have an antihyperlipidemic effect.

Large intakes of nicotinic acid have also been associated with cardiac arrhythmias, increased serum uric acid, itching, nausea, stomach pain, and diarrhea in some individuals (Coronary Drug Project Research Group, 1975). At very high doses, over 3 g/day, niacin may lead to reversible abnormal liver function (Einstein et al., 1975).

Niacin increases blood glucose level (Shansky, 1981), and this may be a problem for diabetic patients (Alhadeff et al., 1984). Because of the niacin-induced release of histamine, use of the vitamin may exacerbate cases of peptic ulcer and asthma (Alhadeff et al., 1984).

REFERENCES

Alhadeff, L., Gualtieri, C. T., and Lipton, M. (1984). Toxic effects of water-soluble vitamins. *Nutr. Rev. 42*:33–40.

Angelin, B., Eriksson, M., and Einarsson, K. (1986). Combined treatment with cholestyramine and nicotinic acid in heterozygous familial hypercholesterolaemia: effects on biliary lipid composition. *Eur. J. Clin. Invest. 16*:391–396.

Blankenhorn, D. H., Nessim, S. A., Johnson, R. L., Sanmarco, M. E., Azen, S. P., and Cashin-Hemphill, L. (1987). Beneficial effects of combined colestipol-niacin therapy on coronary atherosclerosis and coronary venous bypass graphs. *J. Am. Med. Assoc. 257*:3233–3240.

Bures, F. A. (1980). Pruritus associated with niacinamide. *J. Am. Acad. Dermatol.* 3:530–531.

Canner, P. L., Berge, K. G., Wenger, N. K., Stamler, J., Friedman, L., Prineas, R. J., and Friedewald, W. (1986). Fifteen year mortality in Coronary Drug Project Patients: long-term benefit with niacin. *J. Am. Coll. Cardiol. 8*:1245–1255.

Carlson, L. A. and Oro, L. (1962). The effect of nicotinic acid on the plasma free fatty acids: demonstration of a metabolic type of sympathicolysis. *Acta Med. Scand. 172*:641–645.

Coronary Drug Project Research Group (1975). Clofibrate and niacin in coronary heart disease. *J. Am. Med. Assoc. 231*:360–381.

Darby, W. J., McNutt, K. W., and Todhunter, E. N. (1975). Niacin. *Nutr. Rev. 33*:289–297.

Einstein, N., Baker, A., Galper, J., and Wolfe, H. (1975). Jaundice due to nicotinic acid therapy. *Am. J. Digest. Dis. 20*:282–286.

Hoeg, J. M., Gregg, R. E., and Brewer, H. B. (1986). An approach to the management of hyperlipoproteinemia. *J. Am. Med. Assoc. 255*: 512–521.

Lees, R. S. and Lees, A. M. (1984). Lipid-lowering drugs: renewed enthusiasm. *Drug Ther. 14*:57–74.

Naito, H. K. (1987). Reducing cardiac deaths with hypolipidemic drugs. *Postgrad. Med. 82*:102–112.

Pattison, A., Eason, C. T., and Bonner, F. W. (1987). Nicotinic acid enhances the production of 6-ketoprostaglandin F1-alpha in human whole blood in vitro. *Res. Commun. Chem. Pathol. Pharmacol. 55*:423–426.

Perry, R. S. (1986). Contemporary recommendations for evaluating and treating hyperlipidemia. *Clin. Pharm. 5*:113–127.

Schaefer, E. J. and Levy, R. I. (1985). Pathogenesis and management of lipoprotein disorders. *N. Engl. J. Med. 312*:1300–1310.

Shansky, A. (1981). Vitamin B3 in the alleviation of hypoglycemia. *Drug and Cosmetic Indust. 129*:68–69, 104–105.

Shepherd, J., Packard, C. J., Patsch, J. R., et al. (1979). Effects of nicotinic acid therapy on plasma high density lipoprotein subfraction distribution and on apolipoprotein A metabolism. *J. Clin. Invest. 63*:858–867.

Smith, S. R. (1981). Severe hypertriglyceridaemia responding to insulin and nicotinic acid therapy. *Postgrad. Med. J. 57*:511–515.

Tikkanen, M. J. and Nikkila, E. A. (1987). Current pharmacologic treatment of elevated Serum Cholesterol. *Circulation 76*:529–533.

Walldius, G. and Wahlberg, G. (1985). Effects of nicotinic acid and its derivatives on lipid metabolism and other metabolic factors related to atherosclerosis. *Adv. Exp. Med. Biol. 183*:281–293.

Weiner, M., Redish, W., and Steele, J. M. (1958). Occurrence of fibrinolytic activity following administration of nicotinic acid. *Proc. Soc. Exp. Biol. Med. 98*:755–757.

Yovos, J. G., Falko, J. M., Patel, S., Newman, H. A. I., and Hill, D. (1982). Nicotinic acid improves lipoprotein profiles and very low density lipoprotein (VLDL) apo C subspecies in types IIA, IIB, and IV hyperlipoproteinemia (HLP). *Clin. Res. 30*:407A.

10

Vitamin B$_{12}$

S. K. Gaby and A. Bendich

I. INTRODUCTION

Vitamin B$_{12}$ is the term used to describe a group of cobalamins, all of which are water-soluble and found almost exclusively in foods of animal origin. The U. S. recommended daily allowance (U.S. RDA) for vitamin B$_{12}$ is 6 µg. Vitamin B$_{12}$ is essential for the functioning of enzymes involved in amino acid, fatty acid, and nucleic acid metabolism. Vitamin B$_{12}$ is also required in the metabolism of folate. A deficiency of vitamin B$_{12}$ causes macrocytic anemia. Deficiency causes degeneration of spinal cord myelin, which leads ultimately to irreversible neural damage and death. Although anemia has traditionally been regarded as the first sign of vitamin B$_{12}$ deficiency, neuropsychiatric disorders that respond to vitamin B$_{12}$ treatment have been reported in the absence of hematological signs of deficiency (Lindenbaum et al., 1988).

A gastric protein, intrinsic factor, is required for absorption of the vitamin. Autoimmune destruction of parietal cells that produce intrinsic factor causes pernicious anemia and requires the use of vitamin B$_{12}$ injections, since there is no absorption of oral vitamin B$_{12}$. Pernicious anemia is fairly common, occurring in about 1–2 persons per 1000 (McIntyre et al., 1959).

Three serum transport proteins (transcobalamin I, II, and III) carry vitamin B$_{12}$. The vitamin is primarily stored in the liver.

Some individuals with gastric disease may have poor absorption of vitamin B_{12} if it is in food, but not if the vitamin is in crystalline (supplement) form (Doscherholmen and Swaim, 1973). These individuals therefore test negative for pernicious anemia (when a supplement is given), yet have a poor vitamin B_{12} status. In a recent study, 60% of a group of patients with gastric disease who also had neurological, cerebral or psychiatric abnormalities were found to have malabsorption of dietary vitamin B_{12} (Carmel et al., 1988). Acute, severe vitamin B_{12} deficiency may also result from excessive exposure to nitrous oxide (Roe, 1985).

Vitamin B_{12} deficiency is relatively common among the elderly (Carethers, 1988), and is associated with neuropsychiatric abnormalities. However, in other studies healthy, noninstitutionalized older people were found to have a vitamin B_{12} status similar to that of younger adults (Hitzhusen et al., 1986). Marginal vitamin B_{12} status appears to be a problem for all individuals with gastritis (Nilsson-Ehle et al., 1989) and for those with achlorhydria, conditions common among the elderly.

II. HEALTH BENEFITS

A. Cancer Chemoprevention

Experimental work with mice suggests that methyl-vitamin B_{12} may be a tumor suppressor (Shimizu et al., 1987). There is some evidence that vitamin B_{12} may also play a role in the prevention of carcinogenesis in humans. Individuals with pernicious anemia and abnormalities in gastric morphology have a significantly higher rate of gastric cancer, as well as a higher incidence of cancers of the buccal cavity and pharynx (Brinton et al., 1989). Although pernicious anemia is treated with vitamin B_{12} injections, latency to diagnosis may be a considerable period (5–7 years), during which vitamin status may be marginal.

A recent intervention trial showed that heavy smokers supplemented with a combination of vitamin B_{12} and folate had significantly decreased precancerous bronchial squamous metaplasia compared to those given placebo treatment (Heimburger et al., 1988). Individuals enrolled in this study were not deficient in either nutrient, and treated subjects received 500 µg of vitamin B_{12} (8333% of U.S. RDA) daily for 4 months.

Circumstantial evidence suggests a possible chemopreventive effect of vitamin B_{12}, which may be secondary to a sparing effect on folic acid. Given the critical role of vitamin B_{12} in DNA synthesis, however, a direct effect of the nutrient on initiation and/or proliferation is plausible.

B. Immune Function

Because pernicious anemia is an autoimmune disease, it is associated with specific immune system changes (Gogos et al., 1986). Tuberculin skin tests, which are positive in individuals with normal immune systems, were changed from negative to positive in five of seven subjects treated with vitamin B$_{12}$ for pernicious anemia (Katka, 1984). Vitamin B$_{12}$ deficiency itself may result in depression of certain immune functions (Bendich and Cohen, 1988).

C. Cardiovascular Health

Vitamin B$_{12}$ is required for the methylation of homocysteine to methionine. In vitamin B$_{12}$ deficiency there is an accumulation of homocysteine. Individuals with congenital defects of vitamin B$_{12}$ metabolism have high homocysteine levels (Chu and Hall, 1988). Homocysteinemia has been shown to cause arteriosclerosis in animals (McCully, 1975) and may increase the risk of cardiovascular disease in humans (McCully, 1969; Kang et al., 1986; see Chapters 7 and 8, "Vitamin B$_6$" and "Folic Acid").

Individuals considered to be at high risk for coronary heart disease were found to have significantly higher levels of plasma free homocysteine than subjects considered to be at low risk (Swift and Shultz, 1986); plasma free homocysteine was found to be negatively correlated with plasma vitamin B$_{12}$.

It has been postulated that vitamin B$_{12}$, as well as other nutrients involved in homocysteine metabolism, might be useful intervention agents in reducing the risk of cardiovascular disease in some individuals. A controlled intervention trial was conducted with 22 subjects who had survived a myocardial infarct (Olszewski et al., 1989). Treated subjects received 300 µg of vitamin B$_{12}$ (with intrinsic factor) daily for 1 week, plus vitamin B$_6$, folate, choline, riboflavin, and troxerutin (an antioxidant flavenoid). This treatment was associated with a decline of serum homocysteine of about 32%, as well as significant reductions in blood total cholesterol, triglycerides, and low-density lipoproteins. There was no change in the control group of 10 untreated subjects and no effect on high-density lipoproteins in either group. Unfortunately, vitamin status before or after supplementation was not reported. The effect of vitamin B$_{12}$ supplementation alone in reducing homocysteinemia has yet to be elucidated.

III. SAFETY

There have been no reported health problems associated with intakes of vitamin B$_{12}$ in excess of 1000 times the U.S. RDA level, except in rare cases of an allergic reaction (Omaye, 1984). Vitamin B_{12} has not been found to be carcinogenic, mutagenic (Environment Mutagen Information Center, 1973), or teratogenic (Richardson and Brock, 1956).

IV. SUMMARY

Marginal deficiency of vitamin B_{12}, particularly in the elderly, may result in neuropsychiatric disorders responsive to supplementation of the vitamin. In addition, frank deficiency leads to macrocytic anemia.

Preliminary studies indicate that vitamin B_{12} may play a role in cancer prevention.

Vitamin B_{12} deficiency is associated with depression of certain immune system functions.

Several studies suggest that vitamin B_{12}, along with folic acid and vitamin B_6, may be protective against cardiovascular disease by reducing blood homocysteine levels.

REFERENCES

Bendich, A. and Cohen, M. (1988). B vitamins: effects on specific and nonspecific immune responses. In *Nutrition and Immunology*, R. K. Chandra, (Ed.). Alan R. Liss, New York, pp. 101–123.

Brinton, L. A., Gridley, G., Hrubec, Z., Hoover, R., and Fraumeni, J. F., Jr. (1989). Cancer risk following pernicious anemia. *Br. J. Cancer 59*: 810–813.

Carethers, M. (1988). Diagnosing vitamin B_{12} deficiency, a common geriatric disorder. *Geriatrics 43*:89–112.

Carmel, R., Sinow, R. M., Siegel, M. E., and Samloff, I. M. (1988). Food cobalamin malabsorption occurs frequently in patients with unexplained low serum cobalamin levels. *Arch. Intern. Med. 148:* 1715–1719.

Chu, R. C. and Hall, C. A. (1988). The total serum homocysteine as an indicator of vitamin B_{12} and folate status. *Am. J. Clin. Pathol. 90*:446–449.

Doscherholmen, A. and Swaim, W. R. (1973). Impaired assimilation of egg Co^{57} vitamin B_{12} in patients with hypochlorhydria and achlorhydria and after gastric resection. *Gastroenterology 64*:913–919.

Gogos, C. A., Kapatais–Zoumbos, K. N., and Zoumbos, N. C. (1986). Lymphocyte subpopulations in megaloblastic anaemia due to vitamin B_{12} deficiency. *Scand. J. Haematol. 37*:316–318.

Heimburger, D. C., Alexander, C. B., Birch, R., Butterworth, C. E., Bailey, W. C., and Krumdieck, C. L. (1988). Improvement in bronchial squamous metaplasia in smokers treated with folate and vitamin B_{12}:

report of a preliminary randomized, double-blind intervention trial. *J. Am. Med. Assoc. 259*:1525–1530.

Hitzhusen, J. C., Taplin, M. E., Stephenson, W. P., and Ansell, J. E. (1986). Vitamin B$_{12}$ levels and age. *Am. J. Clin. Pathol. 85*:32–36.

Kang, S. S., Wong, P. W. K., Cook, H. Y., Norusis, M., and Messer, J. V. (1986). Protein–bound homocyst(e)ine: a possible risk factor for coronary artery disease. *J. Clin. Invest. 77*:1482–1486.

Katka, K. (1984). Immune functions in pernicious anaemia before and during treatment with vitamin B$_{12}$. *Scand. J. Haematol. 32*:76–82.

Lindenbaum, J., Healton, E. B., Savage, D. G., Brust, J. C. M., Garrett, T. J., Podell, E. R., Marcell, P. D., Stabler, S. P., and Allen, R. H. (1988). Neuropsychiatric disorders caused by cobalamin deficiency in the absence of anemia or macrocytosis. *N. Eng. J. Med. 318*:1720–1728.

McCully, K. S. (1969). Vascular pathology of homocysteinemia: implications for the pathogenesis of arteriosclerosis. *Am. J. Pathol. 56*:111–128.

McCully, K. S. (1975). Homocystine, atherosclerosis and thrombosis: implications for oral contraceptive users. *Am. J. Clin. Nutr. 28*:542–549.

McIntyre, P. A., Hahn, R., Conley, C. L., and Glass, B. (1959). Genetic factors in predisposition to pernicious anemia. *Bull. Johns Hopkins Hosp. 104*:309–342.

Nilsson-Ehle, H., Landahl, S., Lindstedt, G., Netterblad, L., Stockbruegger, R., Westin, J., and Ahren, C. (1989). Low serum cobalamin levels in a population study of 70- and 75-year-old subjects: gastrointestinal causes and hematological effects. *Dig. Dis. Sci. 34*:716–723.

Olszewski, A. J., Szostak, W. B., Bialkowska, M., Rudnicki, S., and McCully, K. S. (1989). Reduction of plasma lipid and homocysteine levels by pyridoxine, folate, cobalamin, choline, riboflavin, and troxerutin in atherosclerosis. *Atherosclerosis 75*:1–6.

Omaye, S. T. (1984). Safety of megavitamin therapy. In *Nutritional and Toxicological Aspects of Food Safety*, M. Friedman, (Ed.). Plenum Press, New York, pp. 169–203.

Richardson, L. R. and Brock, R. (1956). Studies of reproduction in rats using large doses of vitamin B12 and highly purified soybean proteins. *J. Nutr. 58*:135–145.

Roe, D. A., (1985) *Drug-Induced Nutritional Deficiencies*, 2nd ed. AVI Publishing Co., Westport, CT, pp. 198–199.

Shimizu, N., Hamazoe, R., Kanayama, H., Maeta, M., and Koga, S. (1987). Experimental study of antitumor effect of methyl–B$_{12}$. *Oncology 44*:169–173.

Swift, M. E. and Schultz, T. D. (1986). Relationship of vitamins B$_6$ and B$_{12}$ to homocysteine levels: risk for coronary heart disease. *Nutr. Rep. Int. 34*:1–14.

Multivitamin Supplements

S. K. Gaby and L. J. Machlin

A small number of well-controlled studies have been conducted to investigate the health benefits of multivitamin supplementation. Summaries of studies demonstrating a benefit from multivitamin/mineral supplementation are given in Table 1.

I. CANCER RISK

Between different geographical areas, and even within countries, there are clusters of individuals who have either a significantly higher or lower incidence of certain types of cancer compared with the general population. This supports the hypothesis that cultural and environmental factors (as well as genetic factors) are important in identifying the etiology of some types of cancer. In comparison with other countries, Australia has a high incidence of colorectal cancer. A study was conducted in Melbourne, Australia, to relate dietary factors to the risk of developing or dying from colorectal cancer (Kune and Kune, 1987). The researchers interviewed 715 people with colorectal cancer and 727 controls who were matched for age and sex. They collected information on individuals' diets for the previous 20 years. The data were consistent with local per capita food consumption figures for that period. The study showed that regular multivitamin supplement intake, independent of dietary factors, had a protective effect against colorectal cancer in this population. The risk for non-users of de-

Table 1 Summary of Studies Demonstrating Benefits of Multivitamin Supplementation

Subjects	Multivitamin	Type of Study	Findings	Reference
Pregnant women with previous NTD pregnancy in Britain	40–100% of U.S. RDA	Open intervention	Supplementation was associated with a reduction in the recurrence of neural tube defect–affected pregnancy	Smithells et al., 1983
Adults in Melbourne	Any kind	Retrospective case-control	The risk of developing colorectal cancer was about 3 times higher in persons who did not use a multivitamin regularly	Kune and Kune, 1987
12– and 13–year-olds in Wales	25–1000% of RDA	Double–blind placebo controlled	Supplement use associated with increased scores on a test of nonverbal intelligence	Benton and Roberts, 1988
Healthy elderly in Newark, NJ	100–200% of U.S. RDA	Intervention	Supplementation was associated with improved in vitro reponse to PHA and improved delayed dermal hypersensitivity	Bogden et al., 1988
Pregnant women in Atlanta	Any kind 3 times a week or more	Retrospective case-control	The risk of having an NTD–affected baby was 2 times higher in women who did not use a periconceptional multivitamin supplement	Mulinare et al.,1988
Healthy elderly in Zagreb	100–200% of U.S. RDA	Double-blind placebo controlled	Supplementation was associated with improved delayed dermal hypersensitivity	Suboticanec et al.,1989

veloping this type of cancer was about 3 times higher than the risk among multivitamin supplement users.

II. NONVERBAL COGNITION

Benton and Roberts (1988) gave a multivitamin-mineral supplement for 8 months to 30 Welsh schoolchildren (12– and 13–year–olds) who had been obtaining micronutrients from their diets at close to recommended daily allowance (RDA) levels. Thirty of their classmates with similar diets received placebos, and 30 took no pills. The group taking the supplement had significantly increased scores on a test of nonverbal intelligence compared to both control groups. The supplement provided most vitamins in amounts well above U.S. RDA levels. (Table 2 shows the vitamin content of the supplement and the RDA for males 11–14 years old; the RDA for females is slightly lower for vitamin A, thiamine, riboflavin, and niacin.)

Many micronutrients, notably the B vitamins, are important for normal brain activity. It has not been shown, however, that quantities of these vitamins in excess of that required to prevent deficiencies will provide any improvement in thinking ability. The results of this study may reflect the correction of a subclinical deficiency of individual nutrients, although the diets did provide close to RDA levels of these nutrients. The authors suggest, for example, that improved cognition may be related to thiamine re-

Table 2   Vitamin Content of Multivitamin-Mineral Supplement Given to Welsh Schoolchildren and RDA[a]

Vitamin	Amount in supplement[a]	RDA for males 11–14 years[b]	% of RDA
Vitamin A	375 µg	1000 µg	37.5
Thiamine	3.9 mg	1.4 mg	278.6
Riboflavin	5 mg	1.6 mg	312.5
Niacin	50 mg	18 mg	277.8
Vitamin B$_6$	12mg	1.8 mg	666.7
Vitamin B$_{12}$	10 µg	3.0 µg	333.3
Vitamin C	500 mg	50 mg	1000
Vitamin D	3 µg	10 µg	30
Vitamin E	70 IU	12 IU	583.3
Folic acid	100 µg	400 µg	25

[a]From Benton and Roberts (1988).
[b]Committee on Dietary Allowance Food and Nutrition Board: *Recommended Dietary Allowances*, 9th rev. ed. Washington, DC, 1980.

pletion (Harrell,1946).   There may also be synergism or an effect due to a generally improved nutritional status.

III. BIRTH DEFECTS

Inadequate nutrition during gestation may be associated with human birth defects. Supplementation with a multivitamin was associated with a significant reduction in the recurrence of neural tube defect (NTD) pregnancies among women who had previously had an NTD-affected infant (Smithells et al., 1983). Maternal multivitamin supplementation also reduced the recurrence of cleft palate/cleft lip in babies with siblings having this condition (Conway, 1958).

A recent retrospective epidemiological study conducted at the Centers for Disease Control compared periconceptional multivitamin use of the mothers of 347 babies with birth defects and mothers of 2829 babies without birth defects in the Atlanta, Georgia, metropolitan area (Mulinare et al., 1988). Periconceptional use was defined as supplementation during the 3 months before and the 3 months following conception. The risk of having an NTD-affected pregnancy was 2 1/2 times higher in the women who did not use a multivitamin supplement during the periconceptional period as compared to those who used a supplement at least 3 times per week (Mulinare et al., 1988).

IV. IMMUNE RESPONSE

A study of the effects of zinc supplementation on immune competence in an elderly population was recently conducted (Bogden et al., 1988). One of the measures of immune function was the in vitro lymphocyte response to a mitogen, phytohemagglutinin (PHA). Of the 15 subjects for whom this index was originally low, 14 showed an improvement after 3 months of supplementation with either the treatment (zinc plus a multivitamin) or placebo (the multivitamin only). This suggests a beneficial effect of multivitamin supplementation on PHA-induced lymphocyte proliferation in this group of elderly subjects. The subjects in both groups also showed an increase in delayed dermal hypersensitivity (DDH), another indication of improved immune response with multivitamin supplementation.

One hundred individuals living in homes for the elderly in Zagreb participated in a study of the effects of multivitamin supplementation on grip strength and immune function (Suboticanec et al., 1989). Nutrient intakes from diet averaged below recommended levels, but were considered "normal" and adequate. Some biochemical measures of vitamin status were low in some subjects, although no subjects had any symptoms of a nutrient deficiency. Multivitamin supplementation was associated with a slightly positive effect on grip strength, but this was not significantly different from placebo. There was a significant improvement in DDH in the multivitamin treated group.

V. MULTIVITAMIN SUPPLEMENTS AND DISEASE

The biochemical role of each vitamin is presumably the same whether the vitamin is taken as a constituent of a multivitamin supplement or if it is taken separately. However, with a multivitamin supplement the impact of each individual vitamin is impossible to isolate. It cannot be assumed that all of the essential nutrients are contributing to the measured effect. It is also possible that two or more micronutrients work cooperatively, such that the combined effect exceeds the individual effect. For example, such a synergism may occur between vitamin E and selenium in reducing cancer risk (Salonen et al. 1985), and between some antioxidant nutrients (β–carotene, and vitamins E and C) in reducing the risk of developing cataracts (Jacques et al., 1988).

REFERENCES

Benton, D. and Roberts, G. (1988). Effect of vitamin and mineral supplementation on intelligence of a sample of schoolchildren. *Lancet 1*: 140–143.

Bogden, J. D., Oleske, J. M., Lavenhar, M. A., Munves, E. M., Kemp, F. W., Bruening, K. S., Holding, K. J., Denny, T. N., Guarino, M. A., Krieger, L. M., and Holland, B. K. (1988). Zinc and immunocompetence in elderly people: effects of zinc supplementation for 3 months. *Am. J. Clin. Nutr. 48:*655–663.

Committee on Dietary Allowances, Food and Nutrition Board (1980). Recommended Dietary Allowances, 9th rev. ed. National Academy of Sciences, Washington DC.

Conway, H. (1958). Effect of supplemental vitamin therapy on the limitation of incidence of cleft lip and cleft palate in humans. *Plastic Reconstruct. Surg. 22:*450–453.

Harrell, R. F. (1946). Mental response to added thiamine. *J. Nutr. 31:*283–298.

Jacques, P. F., Chylack, L. T., Jr., McGandy, R. B., and Hartz, S. C. (1988). Antioxidant status in persons with and without senile cataract. *Arch. Opthalmol. 106*: 337–340.

Kune, G. A. and Kune S. (1987). The nutritional causes of colorectal cancer: an introduction to the Melbourne study. *Nutr. Cancer 9:*1–4.

Mulinare, J., Cordero, J. F., Erickson, J. D., and Berry, R. J. (1988). Periconceptional use of multivitamins and the occurrence of neural tube defects. *J. Am. Med. Assoc. 260*:3141–3145.

Salonen, J. T., Salonen, R., Lappetelainen, R., Maenpaa, P. H., Alfthan, G., and Puska, P. (1985). Risk of cancer in relation to serum concentrations of selenium and vitamins A and E: matched case-control analysis of prospective data. *Br. Med. J. 290*:417–420.

Smithells, R. W., Seller, M. J., Harris, R., Fielding, D. W., Schorah, C. J., Nevin, N. C., Sheppard, S., Read, A. P., Walker, S., and Wild, J. (1983). Further experience of vitamin supplementation for prevention of neural tube defect recurrences. *Lancet 1*:1027–1031.

Suboticanec, K., Stavljenic, A., Bilic-Pesic, L., Gorajscan, M., Gorajscan, D., Brubacher, G., and Buzina, R. (1989). Nutritional status, grip strength, and immune function in institutionalized elderly. *Int. J. Vit. Nutr. Res. 59*:20–28.

12

General Summary

This review describes the function of vitamins and health benefits associated with maintaining nutritional status at optimal rather than marginal levels.

A number of surveys of food consumption and/or nutritional status have consistently shown that a significant proportion of the U.S. population is at risk for inadequacy of many important micronutrients. This is particularly true for a number of groups, such as smokers, weight-loss dieters, strict vegetarians, oral contraceptive users, alcohol users, adolescents, pregnant and lactating women, the elderly, diabetics, and individuals with chronic digestive tract disorders. Marginal nutritional status may contribute to the risk of chronic degenerative diseases and cancer. Additionally, there are reports that comparatively high intakes of more than the U.S. Recommended Daily Allowance (RDA) of certain vitamins (dietary or supplemental) are associated with specific health benefits. This suggests that vitamin requirements for optimal health may exceed the U.S. RDA under certain circumstances.

The health benefits of individual vitamins are summarized below.

I. VITAMIN A

There is an association between low retinol intake and increased risk of breast cancer. Vitamin A is effective in the treatment of some precancerous conditions, such as oral leukoplakias and esophageal dysplasia.

High-dose vitamin A supplements reduce morbidity and the incidence of bronchopulmonary dysplasia in premature infants.

Poor vitamin A status is associated with compromised immune system function. The morbidity (particularly blindness) and mortality associated with measles infection in marginally nourished children can be reduced by high-dose supplementation with vitamin A.

Hypervitaminosis A may result from acute ingestion of about 500,000 IU of vitamin A by an adult, or from a chronic daily intake of about 100,000 IU. High intakes (above the U.S. RDA of 8000 IU) should be avoided by pregnant women.

II. β–CAROTENE

Free radical and singlet oxygen-initiated attack of vital cell components, mutations, and immunosuppression have been implicated in the progression of various disorders, including cancers. In experimental models and epidemiological studies, β–carotene is associated with suppression of these potentially harmful processes and enhances immune system function.

The antimutagenic properties of β–carotene have been demonstrated in studies of individuals who chew tobacco and betel nuts.

An overwhelming number of studies have demonstrated that high intake of β–carotene-rich foods is associated with reduced risk of cancer, particularly lung cancer. In epidemiologic studies, a strong association between low β–carotene status/intake and greater cancer risk has been reported for cancer of the bladder, breast, cervix, colon/rectum, esophagus, gastrointestinal tract, lung, oropharynx/head and neck, and stomach (primarily cancers of the squamous cell type). The most significant pattern is that associating higher β–carotene intake/status with lower risk of lung cancer. The reduction in cancer risk appears to be due mainly to β–carotene, not other carotenoids, and to be independent of the provitamin A function of β–carotene.

β–Carotene is an extremely safe substance; daily intakes up to 180 mg have not been associated with any toxicity.

III. VITAMIN D

Vitamin D, a prohormone traditionally classified as a vitamin, is known to be critical for bone maintenance and the absorption and metabolism of calcium and phosphorus.

The elderly, infants, vegetarians, individuals with limited ultraviolet light absorption (due to skin pigmentation and/or sun exposure), and people with certain medical conditions may be at risk of poor vitamin D status.

Epidemiological evidence indicates that adequate vitamin D status can reduce the risk of osteoporosis.

Vitamin D, presumably via calcium metabolism, appears to play some role in regulating blood pressure. Good vitamin D status is associated with reduced risk of hypertension.

There is suggestive, but very preliminary evidence that vitamin D may have an anticarcinogenic function, particularly in colon cancer.

Vitamin D can be very toxic at high intakes. No adverse effects in healthy adults have been reported for consumption up to about 62 times the U.S. RDA. Vitamin D is tetratogenic in animal models; intakes by women of childbearing potential should be limited to U.S. RDA levels.

IV. VITAMIN E

Vitamin E functions in the body as the major lipid–soluble antioxidant, helping to protect lipid membranes against the injurious effects of excessive free radicals.

Generally, individuals who develop cancer have had lower blood levels of vitamin E than control subjects in prospective studies.

Mortality from ischemic heart disease was inversely related to blood vitamin E levels.

Vitamin E supplementation decreases platelet aggregation in diabetic subjects but is not very effective in normal individuals. Supplements of 200 IU/day reduced in vitro platelet activity in women on oral contraceptives and 400 IU/day inhibited in vitro platelet adhesion to collagen in healthy adults. These effects on platelet function suggest a role for vitamin E in the prevention of thrombotic disease.

Children with a high vitamin E status had improved responses to some indices of immune function. Elderly subjects with blood levels of vitamin E over 1.35 mg/dl had fewer infections than those with lower levels. Supplementation with vitamin E improved in vivo and in vitro measures of immune system function in a healthy elderly population.

In a retrospective epidemiological study, consumption of a vitamin E supplement (usually 400 IU/day) reduced the relative risk of developing cataracts.

Heavy exercise is associated with increased lipid peroxidation, and this increase can be moderated by vitamin E supplementation. Study results suggest that vitamin E may help protect against exercise-induced muscle injury.

Administration of 1200 IU/day vitamin E resulted in significant improvement in symptoms of medication-induced tardive dyskinesia.

Based on evidence from a limited number of trials, vitamin E supplementation appears to alleviate anemia in G6PD deficient subjects, and to reduce the proportion of irreversibly sickled red blood cells in sickle cell anemia.

Vitamin E intake at high levels has been found to be safe in human and animal studies, with a low incidence of mild and reversible side effects. Vitamin E supplementation is contraindicated during anticoagulant therapy.

V. VITAMIN C

Adequate vitamin C status is necessary for the formation of collagen, a critical step in wound healing. Vitamin C is an essential nutrient for maintaining healthy bones.

Epidemiological evidence suggests that vitamin C-rich foods may reduce the risk of developing cancers of the gastrointestinal tract.

In vitro and animal studies indicate that vitamin C may have a role in enhancing immune function. Ascorbic acid supplementation has been associated with improvement in certain indices of immune response in human subjects.

Supplemental vitamin C may reduce risk factors for cardiovascular disease by increasing levels of high-density lipoproteins, and by reducing total cholesterol in hyperlipidemic individuals. There is additional, albeit limited evidence that a high intake of vitamin C may be efficacious in reducing blood pressure and inhibiting platelet aggregation, and lowering risk of stroke.

A high vitamin C status has been associated with a reduced risk of cataract development, possibly through a reduction in the oxidative destruction of lens proteins.

Vitamin C improves nonheme iron absorption when both nutrients are present simultaneously in the diet.

There is evidence that adequate intake of vitamin C reduces the risk of periodontal disease. Some recent findings suggest that the level of vitamin C required for optimal periodontal health may be more than the current U.S. RDA.

Earlier evidence of the efficacy of vitamin C in treatment or prevention of the common cold is equivocal. However, many of the studies had serious design flaws. The preliminary report of a recent, well–controlled investigation suggests that high intake of vitamin C may reduce the severity of cold symptoms.

Because adverse effects of oral vitamin C supplementation have not been convincingly demonstrated, even at intakes as high as 10–20 g/day, a safe upper limit can not be defined.

VI. VITAMIN B₆

Vitamin B₆ supplementation significantly reduces the symptoms of carpal tunnel syndrome (CTS) in many patients. CTS may be associated with an increased demand for the vitamin.

Although the reports are controversial, vitamin B₆ supplementation appears to relieve symptoms of premenstrual syndrome in some women.

In preliminary studies, relief of asthmatic symptoms has been associated with vitamin B₆ supplementation.

Preliminary data indicate that vitamin B₆ may play a role in improving immune system function.

Inherited homocystinuria and high circulating homocysteine levels, which are associated with increased risk of atherosclerosis, may respond to vitamin B₆ supplementation.

Very high intakes of vitamin B₆ have been shown to cause sensory neuropathy which is usually reversible. Daily intakes below 500 mg for up to 6 months, however, appear to be safe.

VII. FOLIC ACID

Folic acid and multivitamin supplement use are associated with decreased recurrence of neural tube defects and cleft palate/cleft lip birth defects. Low maternal serum folate levels were associated with a substantially greater incidence of birth defects in infants whose mothers were taking anticonvulsant medication.

Subjects with cervical dysplasia were found to have lower serum folate levels than controls; supplementation with folic acid improved cytology scores of cases. Folic acid supplementation also reduced the number of abnormal (precancerous) bronchial cells in individuals with bronchial squamous metaplasia and the incidence of neoplasia in chronic ulcerative colitis.

Inherited homocystinuria and high circulating homocysteine levels, which are associated with increased risk of atherosclerosis, may respond to folic acid supplementation.

Folic acid is believed to be safe in normal subjects even at intakes as high as 15 mg/day.

VIII. NIACIN

High-dose supplementation of nicotinic acid is a standard therapy for hyperlipidemia and is associated with reduced coronary mortality. Nicotinic acid ingestion at high levels is associated with transient flushing. Prolonged high dose intake may cause liver damage and other adverse effects.

IX. VITAMIN B$_{12}$

Preliminary studies indicate that vitamin B$_{12}$ may play a role in the treatment of precancerous lesions and in cancer prevention.

Vitamin B$_{12}$ deficiency is associated with depression of certain immune system functions.

Inherited homocystinuria and high circulating homocysteine levels, which are associated with increased risk of atherosclerosis, may respond to vitamin B$_{12}$ supplementation.

X. MULTIVITAMIN PREPARATIONS

Studies have found associations between regular multivitamin supplement use and reduced colorectal cancer risk, lower incidence of neural tube birth defects, improved scores of nonverbal cognition, and improved immune function in certain groups of elderly persons.

Index

T - #0129 - 101024 - C0 - 234/156/13 [15] - CB - 9780824783822 - Gloss Lamination